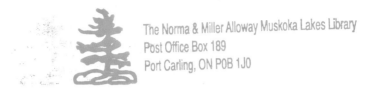
Fat Burning Exercises
For Energy & Weight Loss

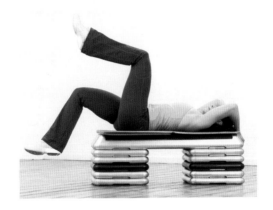

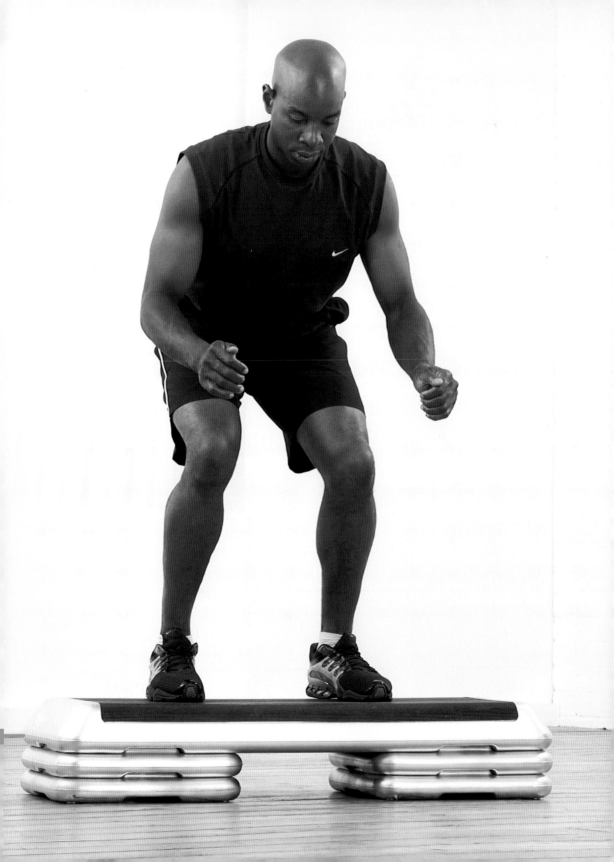

Fat Burning Exercises
For Energy & Weight Loss

A STEP-BY-STEP GUIDE

INCREASE YOUR VITALITY

20-MINUTE WORKOUTS

Jane Wake

Main Street
A division of Sterling Publishing Co., Inc.
New York

Library of Congress Cataloging-in-Publication Data Available

10 9 8 7 6 5 4 3 2 1

Published by Main Street, a division of Sterling Publishing Co., Inc.
387 Park Avenue South, New York, NY 10016
© 2005 by PRC Publishing

An imprint of **Chrysalis** Books Group plc

Distributed in Canada by Sterling Publishing
c/o Canadian Manda Group, 165 Dufferin Street
Toronto, Ontario, Canada M6K 3H6

Printed in China

ISBN 1 4027 1968 X

The exercise programs described in this book are based on well-established
practices proven to be effective for over-all health and fitness, but they are
not a substitute for personalized advice from a qualified practitioner. Always
consult with a qualified health care professional in matters relating to your
health before beginning this or any exercise program. This is especially
important if you are pregnant or nursing, if you are elderly, or if you have
any chronic or recurring medical condition. As with any exercise program,
if at any point during your workout you begin to feel faint, dizzy, or have
physical discomfort, you should stop immediately and consult a physician.

The purpose of this book is to educate and is sold with the
understanding that the author and the publisher shall have neither liability
nor responsibility for any injury caused or alleged to be caused directly
or indirectly by the information contained in this book.

Contents

Introduction

So you want to burn fat? Well you have come to the right book and at the right time, when knowledge about the effects of exercise and how to maximize your fat-burning potential has never been greater.

The idea of fat burning workouts is not entirely new. Since the early 1990s there have been a number of books and countless videos on fat burning. However, many of the claims they made were not substantiated by scientific evidence and some advice was proven later to be wholly misguided.

There was a time, for example, when people were told that the best way to burn fat was to sit on an exercise bike on the easiest resistance level and stay there for two hours, barely working up a sweat. The idea was based on an unfortunate misunderstanding about how the body used and stored fat. Rather then make people lose weight, it had a tendency to make them fatter!

How you burn fat

In order for your body to function you need to burn fuel, derived in the main from a mixture of carbohydrate and fats in the food you eat. Fat is often viewed as a reserve fuel, carbohydrates being the most preferred energy source for your body, from brain function to muscle activity. It is often thought, therefore, that you burn carbohydrate first and then your body switches to using fat reserves. Research has proven, however, that we do in fact burn a mixture of both of these fuel sources together. When you place extra demands on your body, more carbohydrate is indeed called upon to help with the extra workload than fat. But you will burn increased amounts of fuel from both sources. Prolonged exercise (over an hour) has been

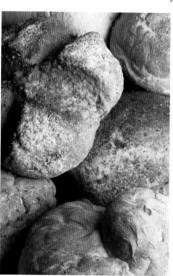 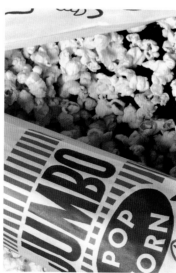 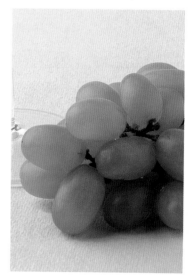

shown to be more effective at burning fat than short bursts of intense activity. The key to success, however, is the overall amount of energy you use. Working at very low levels for long periods of time may start to utilize more fat as a fuel source but at a very slow rate. If you think of this energy as food calories (Kcal), you could burn, say, an additional 100 calories in an hour with a low intensity activity, (in addition, that is, to your normal, or resting, metabolic rate). Low level exercise therefore may not actually burn enough energy to compensate for the amount of energy you consume, leading to weight gain. One small chocolate chip cookie (1 oz) has around 120 calories. If you only burn up an additional 100 calories through exercise, then you will store the excess 20 calories as fat. But there is no point trying to work at really high intensities to burn 600 calories an hour, if it's so hard that you give up after 10 minutes, burning the same, negligible 100 additional calories.

People who have a higher proportion of muscle in their body will burn fuels at a higher rate than those with lower levels of lean muscle tissue, that is, they have a higher resting metabolic rate. They need more fuel simply to function, to stay alive, for breathing, maintaining body temperature, and digesting food. Whatever your body's

makeup, the process of exercising regularly and being fit will boost your metabolism, causing you to burn more fat even when at rest!

So to burn fat you need to:

- Exercise at a level at which your overall energy expenditure is more than the amount of energy in the food you consume.

- Exercise with a view to being able to keep going for a reasonable length of time.

- Do exercises that will help to increase your lean muscle tissue.

- Exercise regularly enough to affect your overall metabolism.

The exercises and workouts in this book are designed to follow these four fat burning guidelines to maximum effect. The book also takes into consideration varying fitness levels, whether you are a complete beginner or a seasoned exerciser. It is not only fat reduction that you will benefit from by following this regime: through the various workouts you will also gain increased strength, better body tone, and improved

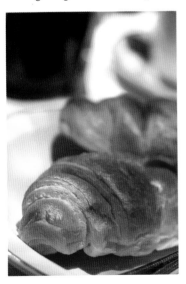
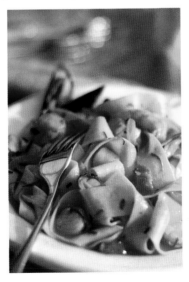
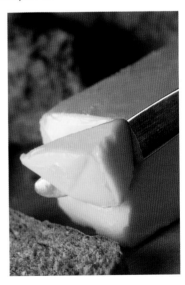

cardiovascular fitness. By performing the "core" exercises you will also gain improvements in posture and a consequent reduction in the general aches and pains that bad posture generates.

How to get the most from your workouts

Start at the right level. If you are not sure, always start with the beginner workouts and then, if you feel this is too easy, progress to the more advanced versions. Sticking to a new exercise regime can be tough at first, but with the right determination and the right support, you can do it!

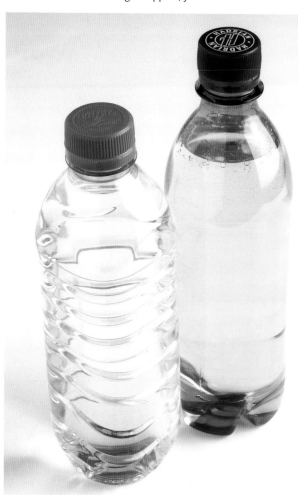

To help you get started:

- Read this book in its entirety first.
- Next, practice the core exercises.
- Then plan your workouts in your diary. From the beginning, tick them off each time you complete them.

Some people find that exercising with a friend or family member helps to them keep going. Setting yourself a new goal each week can also help, such as learning a new exercise or increasing the intensity levels. If you do not feel like exercising, keep reminding yourself that it is *regular* workouts that will get you results—and also how great you'll feel once you have followed through!

Safety and technique

Always follow the advice given on safety, technique, and correct intensity levels. Exercise is only worth doing if you are going to do it right. Use poor techniques—such as using your back in the wrong way in an exercise, or working at the wrong level of intensity—and you will become frustrated at your lack of ability and progress and give up, or injure yourself.

If you have any injury concerns, are pregnant, or unwell, you should consult with your medical practitioner before starting a new exercise program.

The exercises are designed for healthy adults. If you are unsure about any aspect of your health, it is recommended that you seek advice from your medical practitioner before you begin.

Always use the correct posture throughout each exercise. To do this you need to be able to hold your spine in its natural curves, using the muscles around it to maintain position. The muscles that do this are called your "core muscles." Exercises targeted at these muscles are provided. By going through the core muscle exercises in this book and continuing to practice them with every workout, you will automatically start to learn correct posture, which is essential for safe technique.

Always follow the guidelines on warming up and cooling down—doing so will prolong your ability to work out, make your exercise safe, and increase your fat-burning potential.

Eight Golden Rules

• Follow exercise instructions carefully. Working out in front of a mirror can be helpful at first. You can check that your body is in the same position as in the photograph.

• Always begin very slowly with each new exercise. You can speed up later, so long as you can maintain your posture and perform the movement as shown. Never swing, heave, or throw yourself into a position.

• Try to concentrate on the muscles you are using, focussing on how your body feels. The exercise Hints & Tips will help you with this.

• Breathe continuously throughout each exercise, aiming to breathe out when you exert most pressure, lifting, pushing, or pressing through a movement.

• Never exercise to extremes, follow the guidelines on intensity carefully. (See following page.)

• Avoid following the same workout on consecutive days. It is important to give variety to your movements and rest periods. Always have at least one or two days of complete rest per week. If you are worried about losing focus, just do some very gentle stretching exercises on your days off.

• Aim to eat $1^1/_2$ to 2 hours before your workout. Research has shown that having a meal or healthy snack before you train will actually improve your performance and help you to burn more calories. If you do not have time to eat, for example, first thing in the morning, eat a light, healthy snack such as a banana at least a half-hour before exercising.

• Water is your lifeline. Not drinking enough will impair your ability to work out and function throughout your day. Aim to drink 3 to 5 pints (1.5 to 2.5 liters) of water a day, sipping plenty before, during, and after your workout.

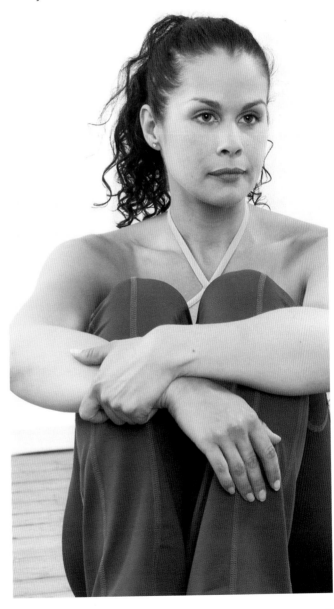

Working at the right intensity

In order to fulfill the four criteria for successful fat burning as outlined on page 7, you need to have a clear idea of what intensity to work at. The key is to exercise at a level that you can manage, but where you feel challenged.

• Think of a scale from 0–10, 0 being rest, 10 being exhaustion. Your aim is to work between 4–6 on this scale, that is, not between 0–3 where it feels so easy that you feel you could keep going for ever, but not 7 or above where it feels too hard to keep going for more than an ineffectually short time. Four to 6 is your fat-burning intensity zone.

• After your warm-up, you should feel your body temperature has risen. During the following 5 minutes, increase the intensity gradually, so that eventually you can feel yourself begin to sweat and your breathing getting heavy. Only you can establish the

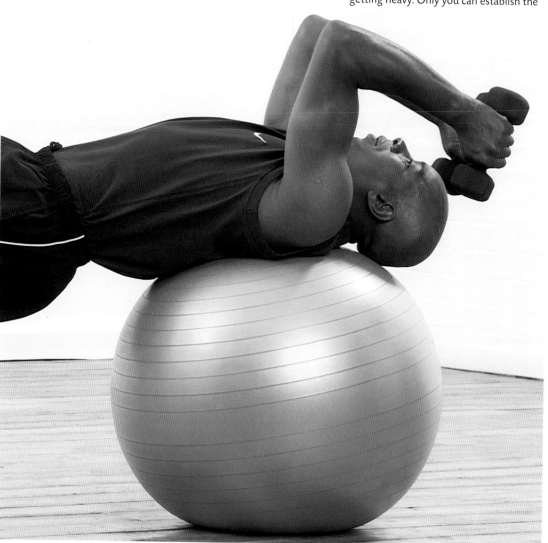

rate you work over the 5 minutes to get to this point, by getting to know your body, and by trial and error.

- Once you are at this level, aim to stay up there. A good test is to see if you can string a sentence together, so try singing one line of a song: if you can, then you are working out at about the right level. If you can sing the whole song, then you are not working hard enough!

- Your aim is to find a level where you can keep going for a minimum of 20 minutes, following your warm-up and including the first 5 minutes. At first you will find it hard to find that level, but the more that you work out, the more in-tune with your body you become, and the easier it will be to find your personal limitations and then approach them, without exceeding them .

- One exception to these intensity guidelines are the interval workouts. For these you will aim to do short bursts of higher intensity training (say, 7 on the above scale) followed by short periods of low intensity training. For this, during your high intensity burst, you should aim to work as hard as you can in the time given. But you must then be able to recover from this high intensity bout of exercise during the low intensity period. If you are not able to recover in that time, then your high bursts of activity need to be done at a slightly lower level.

Above all remember: to maximize your fat burning potential, you have to work out as hard as you can, but over the full 20 minutes.

How to warm up and cool down effectively

The Warm-up
The most effective way to warm up is do the same exercises that are in your chosen workout but at a much lower intensity. If you are going out for a walk, it's simple, just start off at a slow, easy pace and gradually increase speed until you feel that you are going into the intensity zones as described. If you are short on time, 5 minutes is your minimum warm-up. If you have longer, then utilize this time with a more gradual warm-up. The longer you give your body to warm up, the better both mentally and physically you will feel to tackle your workout. Each of the workouts has its own warm-up, which mimics the first exercise in your workout but at a much lower intensity.

You need to ensure that your muscles have been warmed up thoroughly—right through to the joint areas. Traditionally, "static" stretches have been used to do this—extending the limbs and holding that position—but research has found that gradually increasing your range of movements to work closer and closer to the joints as you warm up is more effective. This is sometimes called "dynamic stretching." To make sure that you have done this effectively I have included some simple dynamic warm-up moves for you to follow with every workout. You will find these on pages 30–35.

The Cool-down
Cooling down is important because it enables your body to recover from your workout, preventing (or reducing) stiffness and lessening the potential for injury. It is also important psychologically, giving you time to relax and enjoy some calm. To cool down, you need to gradually decrease your intensity over 3 minutes, bringing yourself out of your intensity zone. Each workout therefore finishes with a slightly lower intensity exercise that will enable you to do this. If, however, after doing the last exercise you feel your heart is still racing, walk around slowly for a further 2 minutes, taking slow, deep breaths.

Follow this with some cool-down stretches. These are extremely important for balancing your workouts, helping to increase your flexibility, muscle balance, and efficiency. You will find these stretches on pages 108–123.

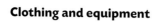

Clothing and equipment

Clothing

It is important to wear comfortable sportswear that allows your skin to breathe as you work out. Most good sports clothes are now made with a material that has special fibers which keep the body cool by taking the sweat away and dispersing it. Avoid simple cottons, which tend to get drenched with sweat, leaving your clothing heavy, damp, and cold next to your skin. The sportswear should not have seams or any roughness that could cause chaffing. Be particularly careful about your inner thigh, underarm, and around the chest and waist.

Women really should wear a sports bra, whatever their size! Go to a specialist shop and have a bra fitted—it is certainly a worthwhile investment that could save you a lot of discomfort.

Wear a supportive sports training shoe. As you will be primarily working inside, go for a cross-training or in-studio shoe that does not have a heavy tread and allows your foot to move on the floor surface, but with enough traction to prevent slipping. If you are to include walking and running as part of your fat-burning activities, invest in an outdoor running shoe. Go to a specialist sport shoe shop for further advice.

Equipment

For the workouts you will need the following equipment. All of these items ae readily available from sports shops and on-line. If you can, try to go to a store so that you can test out the equipment before you purchase.

Exercise ball Sometimes called a Swiss ball, stability ball, or fit ball. This will usually need to be about 17, 21, or 26 inches in diameter, depending on your leg length. It is important to work with a ball that has been fully inflated. Flat balls put you into the wrong height positions and lower the effectiveness of your exercises. Make sure you can purchase a pump with your ball or have access to one that works with the valve. Some balls come in slightly smaller sizes, some much larger, but the latter are not for our kind of exercises. Here is an approximate guide:

- If you are less than 5 ft. 3 in., use a 17-in. ball.
- If you are 5 ft. 3 in. to 5 ft. 8 in., use a 21-in. ball.
- If you are taller than 5 ft. 8 in., use a 26-in. ball.

And so on: the taller you are, then of course the bigger the ball required. For a more accurate guide, sit on a ball with your back tall and your pelvis on the center of the ball. Your knees should be bent comfortably at about a 90 degree angle.

Exercise tube or band For ease and comfort it is recommended that you work with a band that has handles at both ends. These latex bands come in different strengths of resistance. You will need to purchase two bands: one for lighter resistance, one for heavier use. If you are a beginner, go for light and medium resistance and if you are more advanced, but have never used bands, then test before you buy.

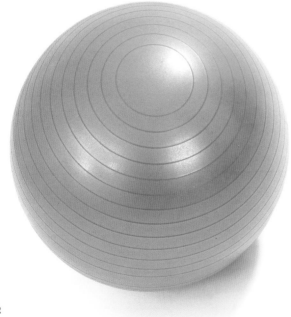

Step or box, adjustable for height You can either purchase an adjustable fitness step or use two sturdy boxes with a minimum top surface area of 12 by 30 inches. They must be made of a pliable but strong material, enough to carry your body weight, and have rubber under-surfaces to prevent slipping. While not being adjustable, your stairs or steps at home will work for most exercises. Beginners and those 5 ft. 3 in. and below should use a step 6–12 inches in height, the more advanced and those 5 ft. 4 in. and above should use one of 8–16 inches.

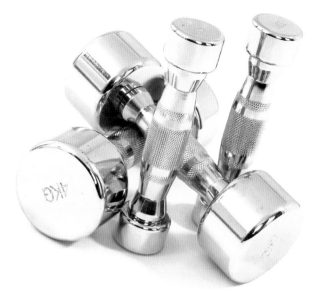

A three-pair set of dumbbells or one pair of adjustable dumbbells If using adjustable dumbbells, make sure that the disk weights fit smoothly on to the bars and that the locks hold tight. Rubber disk weights with metal spin locks are the safest to use, but they tend to be more expensive, so try before your buy. Beginners should work with weights between 2–8 lb. and the more advanced with 5–15 lb.

You will also need a towel or mat to lie on, an additional towel to help with certain stretches and exercises, plus a stopwatch, or at least a watch with a second hand.

How to plan your workouts

You have a number of different workouts to choose from. Planning them, and planning an order to do them, is an important part of your routine. Remember that it is regularity of effort that will get you the best results, so get your diary out now and make some dates with your fat burner book. You have 8 workouts to choose from, plus running or power-walking sessions as alternatives. This really does give longevity and versatility to the workout regime, enabling you to choose workouts that suit you best. For example, if you prefer to be outside, or the weather's particularly good, substitute some of your indoor workouts for outdoor alternatives.

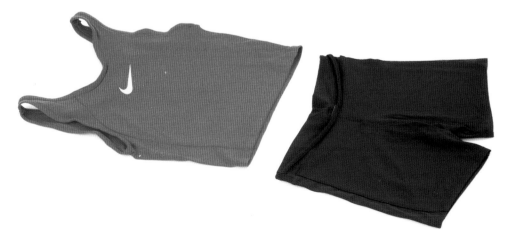

It is worth remembering that variety in your fitness training can be beneficial in your efforts to burn fat. Have you ever heard of the "plateau" effect? This is what happens if you do not progress your training and do the same exercises, month after month. Our bodies learn to adapt to the exercise to such an extent that we start to burn less calories. So as well as ensuring that you are doing workouts to suit you, remember that after your first initial eight weeks, you must continue to lengthen your workouts and/or use alternatives. For example, if you have never power-walked or run before, try either as a substitute for one of your cardio circuits.

Here is an eight-week plan example. If you feel unsure about making up you own plan, then begin with this one.

Week 1 A minimum of 3 workouts. To include 2 cardio circuit workouts and 1 strength workout.

Week 2 A minimum of 4 workouts. This needs 2 cardio circuits, 1 interval session, and 1 strength workout.

Week 3 Six workouts. To include 2 cardio circuits, 1 interval session, 1 strength workout, 1 Mix It session, and 1 Core Strength And Length session. Your Core Strength And Length session can be completed on the same day as one of your other workouts.

Week 4 onward Continue with your 6 x 20-minutes workouts as in week 3. However, aim to lengthen one of your cardio circuits by 3–6 minutes each week by going back and repeating the circuit exercises. For example, on week 4, repeat exercise 1 and 2, on week 5 repeat exercises 1, 2, and 3, on week 6 repeat exercise 1, 2, 3, and 4. Keep doing this until you have repeated all the exercises, to give you one 40-minute workout. As you get fitter, you can also do the same with your other cardio circuit and interval sessions.

You must do this gradually, just 3–6 minutes, that's one or two exercises added to each workout each week. Doing this will not only burn more fat, it will increase your ability to burn fat.

On page 16 is an eight-week example which progresses at the quickest rate. You could copy this one into your diary. But remember that this is a kind of ideal scenario and may not be suitable for you. And we all live in the

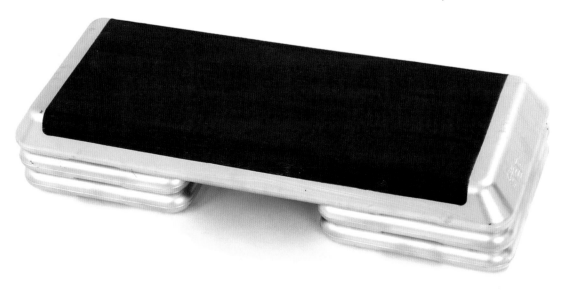

real world—events can conspire against the best laid plans. But the whole workout regime begins with something we all have, even the busiest—20 minutes. Make sure, whatever plan you make, that you monitor your progress by ticking off each session you complete.

If you start missing sessions, then stop and rethink. If the longer workouts are getting too hard to fit in, then continue the shorter workouts for a little longer, until you feel ready to move on.

More frequent workouts that are easier for you to fit in will certainlyt reap more benefits that the odd long session here and there.

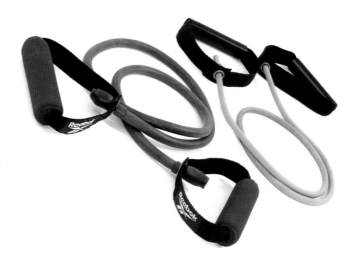

Every little extra helps

We all burn fat at slightly different rates. Some people are genetically geared to have faster metabolisms than others, which can account, in part, for why some of us naturally carry less body fat. But the apparent increase in the numbers of obese people in the developed world is surely down to lifestyle.

Using a fat burner workout program such as this one, and sticking to it, is one way you can change your lifestyle to ensure you do not become unhealthy and overweight. There are, however, a number of other simple steps that you can take not only to improve your health but also to increase your fat-burning potential. No prizes for guessing what is top of the list.

Take a serious look at your diet. As explained earlier in this chapter, it is the deficit between the number of calories that you consume and the number of calories that you burn which results in fat loss. By eating healthily and reducing the number of fat calories you consume, you make the task of losing fat through exercise so much easier. You have read the following before: please read it again and act on it.

• Cut out sugary, fatty junk foods such as cakes and sodas and substitute with fruit, fruit juice, and water instead.

• Cut down on (or better, cut out) foods cooked in fat and grill and steam instead of frying and roasting.

• Aim to have your plate always half-full of vegetables or salad.

• Start eating smaller portions by gradually reducing the amount of food on your plate at each meal.

• Eat three small meals a day, with only healthy snacks in between.

People who fidget tend to burn more calories. While this doesn't mean you should develop irritating habits, generally being more active can help with your fat loss. There are 3,500 calories in a pound of fat. By burning around 100 extra calories a day through general activity, that's an extra pound of fat gone in a month, 12 lb. in a year! To burn an extra 100 calories a day, aim to do a minimum of 30 minutes of increased activity, which can be built up throughout the day at different times.

Choose to climb the stairs rather than taking the elevator, walk 5 minutes or 25 minutes to the grocery store instead of driving, get out and work in the backyard, or do the housework—it all counts.

	MON	TUE	WED	THUR	FRI	SAT	SUN
Week 1	Cardio Circuit x 20 mins	REST	Fat Burner Strength x 20 mins	REST	REST	Cardio Circuit x 20 mins	REST
Week 2	Cardio Circuit x 20 mins	REST	Fat Burner Strength x 20 mins	Interval Session x 20 mins	REST	Cardio Circuit x 20 mins	REST
Week 3	Cardio Circuit x 20 mins	REST	Fat Burner Strength x 20 mins	Interval Session x 20 mins	Core Strength & Length x 20 mins	Cardio Circuit x 20 mins	Fat Burner Mix It x 20 mins
Week 4	Cardio Circuit x 26 mins	REST	Fat Burner Strength x 20 mins	Interval Session x 20 mins	Core Strength & Length x 20 mins	Cardio Circuit x 20 mins	Fat Burner Mix It x 20 mins
Week 5	Cardio Circuit x 32 mins	REST	Fat Burner Strength x 20 mins	Interval Session x 20 mins	Core Strength & Length x 20 mins	Cardio Circuit x 20 mins	Fat Burner Mix It x 20 mins
Week 6	Cardio Circuit x 40 mins	REST	Fat Burner Strength x 20 mins	Interval Session x 20 mins	Core Strength & Length x 20 mins	Cardio Circuit x 20 mins	Fat Burner Mix It x 20 mins
Week 6	Cardio Circuit x 40 mins	REST	Fat Burner Strength x 20 mins	Interval Session x 26 mins	Core Strength & Length x 20 mins	Cardio Circuit x 26 mins	Fat Burner Mix It x 20 mins
Week 7	Cardio Circuit x 40 mins	REST	Fat Burner Strength x 20 mins	Interval Session x 32 mins	Core Strength & Length x 20 mins	Cardio Circuit x 32 mins	Fat Burner Mix It x 20 mins
Week 8	Cardio Circuit x 40 mins	REST	Fat Burner Strength x 20 mins	Interval Session x 40 mins	Core Strength & Length x 20 mins	Cardio Circuit x 40 mins	Fat Burner Mix It x 20 mins

Week 9 onward Continue to vary your plan by substituting at least one workout per week with one of the alternative workouts below.

ALTERNATIVE WORKOUTS

Substitute Cardio Circuits for:–   Power Walking, Running, or Fat Burner Step Circuit
Substitute Interval Sessions for:–   Outdoor Interval Session
Substitute Fat Burner Mix it Session for:– Outdoor Crosstrainer Session

Connecting To Your Core

Your core muscles are the ones that you cannot see. They tend to lie deep within your body: close to the spine and supporting structures such as your pelvis and shoulder areas. They are really important muscles that hold you in correct postural positions. Weak core muscles can lead to back, neck, and shoulder pain and an inability to perform tasks, from exercise to housework. More often than not this is caused by poor lifestyle habits such as incorrect sitting and standing positions or careless movements such as bending your back to lift something from the floor. Learning to connect to your core can really help with every day life as well as improve your exercise technique.

But what has all this got to do with fat burning?
By connecting to your core muscles and generally being more aware of your posture you will start to use more muscle with every action you take. The result? You burn more calories and use up more fat energy stores. This makes the exercise harder but also a lot safer, more efficient, and more effective—worth that little bit of extra effort!

How to connect to your core

There are three main "core" areas to focus on:

Your Deep Abdominal Muscles The main muscle concerned here is called the Tranversus Abdominus. This lies like a corset around your abdomen, between your ribs and pelvis. Learning to use it will help to support your lower back in conjunction with deep back muscles, which lie directly along the spine. Just by pulling in gently you can train this muscle to hold continuously. It is also the most effective way to flatten your stomach. To activate these, think of slowly and gently drawing your belly towards your spine.

Your Pelvic Floor These are a series of muscles, which lie like a hammock underneath your pelvis. As well as helping to control movement from your bladder and bowel, they have direct relationship with your Transversus Abdominis (TA)—when you cough or sneeze, for example, you will feel a reflex in your TA muscle, at the same time yourpelvic floor should pull up and tighten. In many of us, this doesn't always happen, the pelvic floor becoming weak in both men and women over time. This is exacerbated in women after childbirth who need to concentrate more on the central part of the pelvic floor. To activate these, think of pulling up underneath you, as if stopping yourself from urinating.

Your Shoulder Girdle There are a number of muscles, both deep and on the surface, that are responsible for supporting your shoulder joint and upper spine. The deepest are a group of muscles called the rotator cuff. These are responsible for holding the shoulder joint in place. Other muscles that lie over the top include your Rhomboids, which work between the shoulder blades and the lower sections of a big muscle called the Trapezius, that act to pull your shoulder blades slightly in and down. If your shoulders tend to round forward and your neck area gets tight and strained, you are going to have a definite weakness in this area.

To activate, think of gently drawing your shoulders back and down. Open your chest area by turning your palms to face forward, bringing your little finger in line with the side seam of your pants. Also aim to lengthen from your ears to your shoulders.

By holding good posture throughout your fat burning routines and by being aware of it in every day activities you will start to activate a greater proportion of muscle in your body, making you stronger, more energized, and more likely to burn fat.

How to hold correct posture

To maintain good posture you need to work the core areas, as described above. Whether doing your fat burner workouts, walking to work, or doing the housework, keep reminding your self of the following points:

• Always keep your back up tall. Lift your chest but at the same time draw your belly in. You should have a small curve in your lower back and back of your neck.

• Ease your shoulders gently back and down. Your shoulders blades should be drawn in flat against the back of your rib cage.

• Draw your chin in without looking down, that is, keep your nose pointing forward.

• Make sure your pelvis is level. Place your hands on your hips and imagine your pelvis is a bucket of water—avoid tipping the water out, front or back. If lying on the floor your pelvis should be level with a small hollow in your lower back.

• Correct posture means maintaining these natural curves using core muscles.

The following exercises will help you to strengthen your core. As well as doing a specific Core Strength and Length workout each week, you will find one of these core exercises in each of your workouts. Your plan should be to practice them every day so that you automatically begin to use your core muscles in everything you do. The more you practice, the more you will connect, and the more calories you will burn!

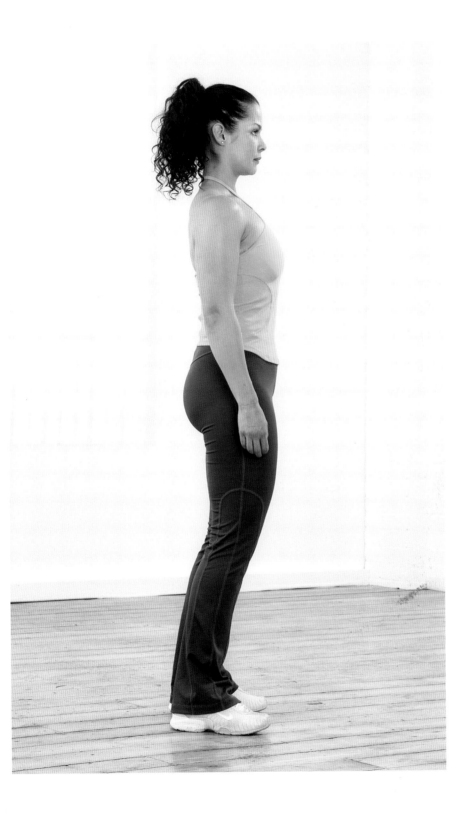

Core Exercises–Beginners

secret squeeze

Aim: To strengthen your pelvic floor muscles situated underneath your pelvis, supporting your lower torso and spine, as well as helping to control your bladder and bowel.
Focus: Concentrate on finding your pelvic floor, deep and close to your abdomen.

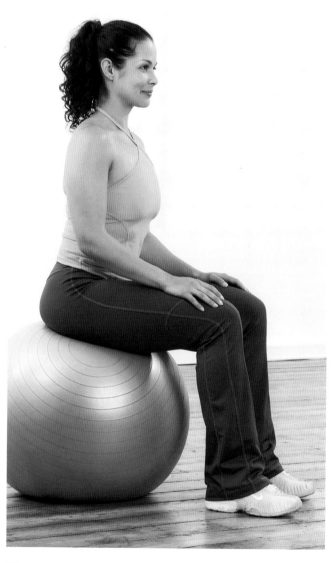

Method

- Sit on your exercise ball. With your back tall; ladies, lean slightly forward, men, stay upright.
- Focus on trying to pull up from inside, as if stopping yourself from urinating.
- Ladies, aim to try to pull up more from the middle; men, simply from front to back.

Hints & Tips

- Don't worry if you can't feel anything at first—keep practicing, but not only when you workout. You can do this exercise anywhere, for example, in the car, at your desk, in the park— wherever you have a seat. Keep repeating it and you will notice the difference.
- To progress: once you have found your pelvic floor muscles, try to do 4–10 slow squeezes, followed by 4–10 quick, fast-firing lifts.

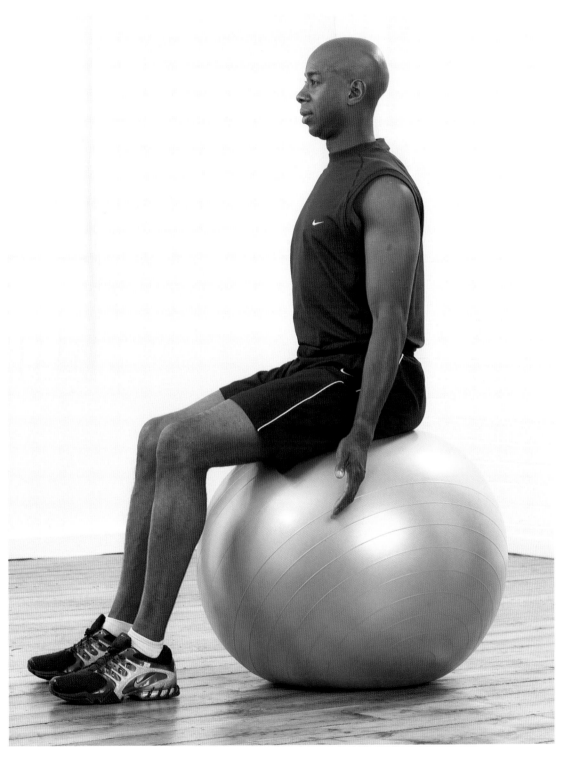

the dumb waiter

Aim: To strengthen and increase awareness of upper back and core shoulder muscles, while lengthening the chest to give better upper body posture.

Focus: Concentrate on holding good posture while focussing on squeezing the muscles that work between your shoulder blades.

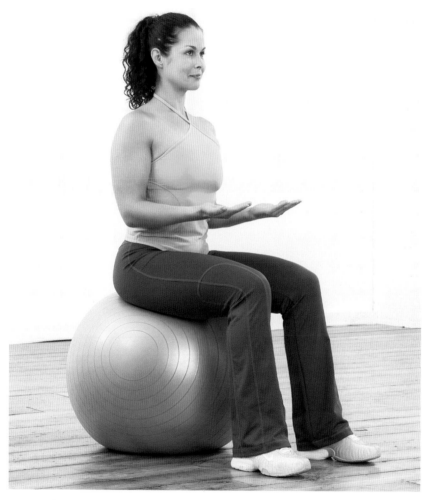

Method

- Sitting tall on your ball, chest lifted, stomach in, and shoulders back and down.
- Place your hands in front of you, elbows bent at 90 degrees, as if carrying a tray. Keeping your elbows close to your ribs, take a breath in and, as you breathe out, squeeze in between your shoulder blades and start to part your hands out to the side.
- Keep drawing your abdomen in toward your spine, with your spine still and tall.

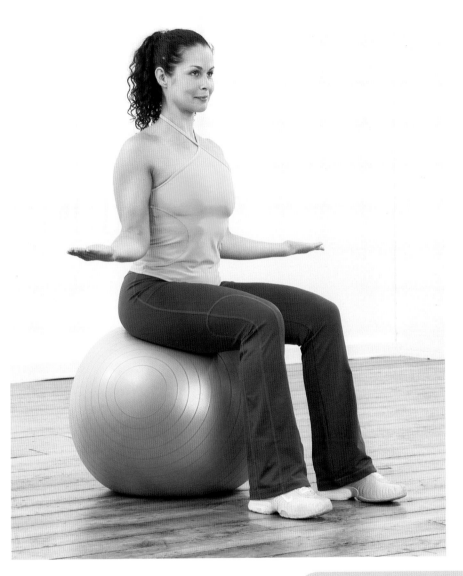

- With your elbows still touching your ribs, hold your hands out to the side for 6 counts, breathing deeply and slowly.
- Lengthen out from the ears to the shoulders, keeping your chin in and the back of your neck long.
- Return to the start and repeat 6–10 times or until your muscles start to become tired.
- To progress, try to complete the exercise while balancing your weight on one leg. This will put extra demands on the TA (core abdominal) muscle and pelvic floor. Use them both to keep you upright.

Hints & Tips

- Remain focused on the shoulder blades—imagine there is a piece of string attached to the bottom of each, drawing them both in and down.
- To ensure that you are pulling back into the right position, check your side profile in a mirror—your shoulder should be pulled back directly to the side with your elbow in line, upper arm vertical.

on all fours

Aim: To prepare for your fat burning exercises, learning to hold abdominals, pelvic floor, and core shoulder muscles stable, while also doing an exercise to work your arms.

Focus: Concentrate on keeping your back completely still, feeling your abs, shoulders, back, and pelvic floor muscles working, as well as the back of your arm muscle (Tricep).

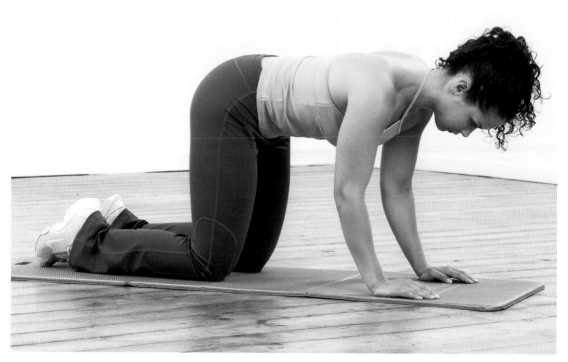

Method

- In an all fours position, make sure your hands are in line with your shoulders, and knees in line with your hips.
- Lift your head by drawing your chin inward—you should be looking down at the floor.
- Draw your shoulders back and down, bring your elbows in, and take your butt back to form a small arch in your lower back.
- Bend your elbows back to lower your upper body.
- Draw your abdomen in to meet your spine and also try to feel your pelvic floor, without changing the position of your back. Keep breathing and hold for 6 counts.

Hints & Tips

- To help you find this position, look in a mirror or use a broom handle as shown above right. The handle should touch the back of your head, between your shoulder blades, and on the base of your spine.
- To progress, try to hold one hand off the floor for 10 slow counts before changing sides.

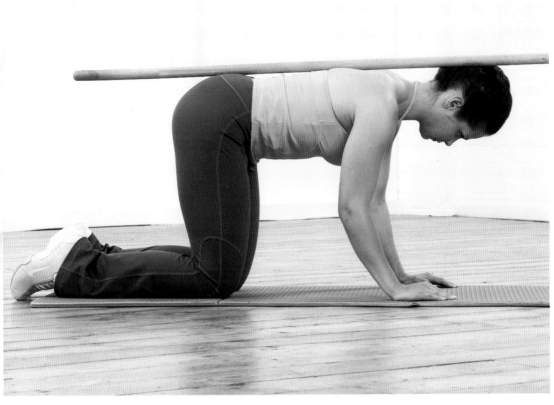

- Once you feel you are stable, try to lift your left hand slightly off the floor.
- Keeping everything level, avoid leaning to your right, and switch hands.
- Your body should feel like it is working intensely, burning extra calories to hold you in the correct position.
- Repeat 6–10 lifts on each hand or until your muscles start to tire.
- Relax by pulling back into a praying position, resting your butt onto your heels.

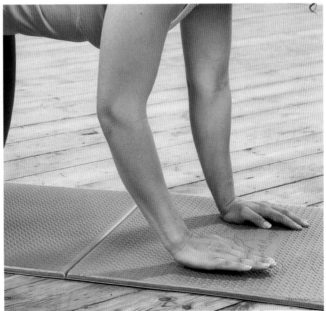

Core Exercises—Advanced

the posture squat

Aim: To establish correct posture for squatting actions, working all your core areas while also toning and strengthening legs (Hamstrings and Quadriceps) and buttock (Gluteus Maximus) muscles.

Focus: Keep checking your back position by looking sideways-on to a mirror.

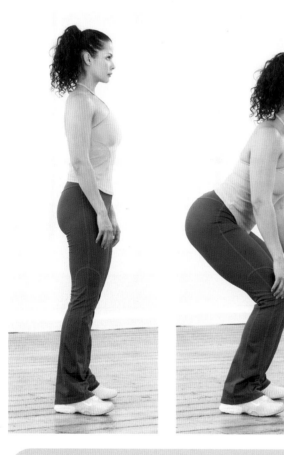

To perform these exercises correctly you must have established how to connect to your pelvic floor, deep abdominal, and deep shoulder and back muscles. If you are not sure, or think you have a weakness in one or more of these areas, do the beginners core exercises instead. Stay with them until you feel you have mastered all core areas, then move onto the advanced moves.

Method

- Place your feet just over hip-width apart, feet turned slightly outward.
- Stand tall, in correct postural alignment. Check your neck, shoulder, lower back, and pelvis positioning (see note about connecting to your core above).
- Take a breath and, as you breathe out, start to bend at your hip and knee joints, sitting your butt out behind you and making sure that your knees don't push forward over your toes.
- Keep slowly lowering, taking deep breaths and re-establishing correct posture and core muscle contraction—you should take at least 4 slow counts to lower.
- When you have gone as far as you comfortably can, going no lower than a 90-degree bend at the knee, take a breath and push back up, taking at least 4 slow counts to lift.
- Re-establishing core muscle connection at the point of lifting is important here. Also, constantly check your back alignment as you lift.
- Repeat 8–12 times or until you start to feel your muscles in your legs and butt tire.

Hints & Tips

- To help you balance, keep your weight into your heels and allow your arms to hang freely forward while still keeping your shoulders back and down.
- Be careful to ensure that you push your weight through your heels and that you connect to your butt muscles as you lift.

the arrow head

Aim: To strengthen and increase awareness of your upper back and core shoulder muscles. Also to work the arms and lengthen the chest to give you better upper body posture.

Focus: Concentrate on your upper back, feeling muscles between your shoulder blades (Rhomboids) working.

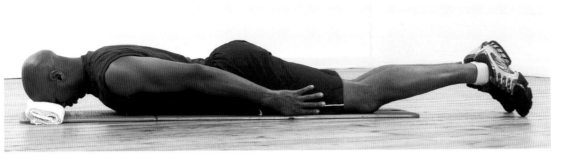

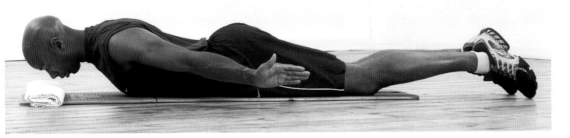

Method

- Lie on your front on the floor, with your forehead resting on a towel and your hands relaxed down by your side.
- Take a breath in and, as you breathe out, lift your abdomen away from the floor, being careful not to lift your hips.
- Draw in through your pelvic floor muscles and start to work your shoulder blades down your back and in toward your spine. Lift your head, neck, and shoulders $1/2$ to 1 inch off the floor. Be careful not to lift any higher because this will place stress on your lower back.
- Now concentrate on the area between your shoulder blades, squeezing them in while rolling your palms in, then out, so that they finish facing out with your thumbs pointing toward the ceiling.
- Recheck that you are using your core abdominal and pelvic muscles.
- Remain looking down at the floor, with the back of your neck long and chin in.
- Hold for another breath, in and out, reconnecting to your core muscles as you breathe out.
- Slowly release back down.
- Repeat 6–10 times or until you feel the muscles in your upper back start to tire.

Hints & Tips

- Make sure that your shoulders are turned out, lengthening through your chest as your arms rotate.
- Aim to create length through your body by also lengthening your arms toward your feet—you should be able to feel the back of your arms contract as you do this.
- Focus on hollowing your midsection and creating length through your body rather than too much lift.
- To progress, hold the position in the second picture for 6–10 slow counts. Continue to breathe, reconnecting to your core as you breathe out.

27

press and lift

Aim: Using your core muscles to keep your back in correct alignment while working arm, chest (Pectoralis Major), and buttock (Gluteus Maximus) muscles.

Focus: Concentrate on the three key core areas to ensure that you keep your back in its natural curves.

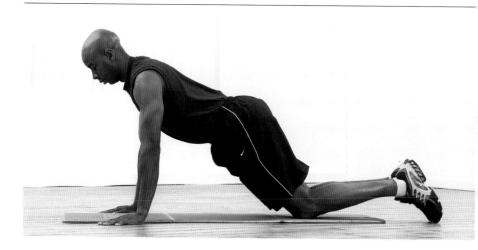

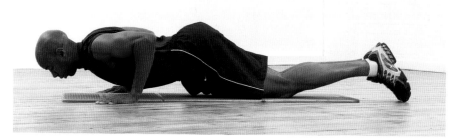

Method

- Go onto your hands and knees, hands at shoulder level, knees positioned together and behind your hips.
- Hold this position and check on your core muscle focus—shoulders drawn back and down with the neck lengthened, nose facing directly down, abdominals pulled in, and pelvic floor muscles connected.
- Slowly lower into a narrow press up position, being careful not to let your back sag or hunch your shoulders. Take at least 4 slow counts to do this.
- Press up, keeping your back still. Take 4 slow counts to lift.
- Hold in your start position; check your core muscle focus.

Hints & Tips

- The most effective way to do this exercise is by using a mirror. At each stage of the exercise stop, hold and check that your lower back, shoulder, and head position are correct.
- To progress, lift one foot off the floor squeezing your butt muscles and lengthening your leg away (see final picture). This is very hard and should only be attempted if you feel you can maintain your core emphasis.

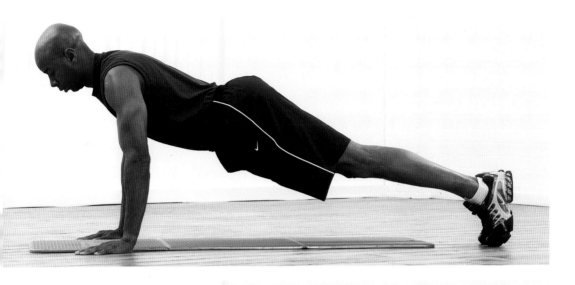

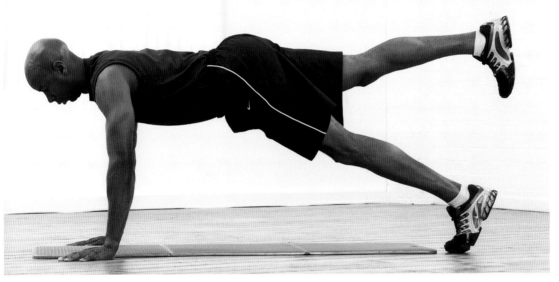

- Now lift into the next stage of the exercise, curling your toes under and pressing back onto the ball of your feet.
- You should be forming a straight plank position with your back at all times—be careful not to stick your butt in the air. Check your position in a mirror.
- Hold here for 4 slow counts. Reconnect again to your core ensuring that you haven't allowed your shoulders to hunch, head to drop, or back to sag.
- Slowly drop to your knees, making sure you maintain your back's natural curves.
- Repeat 2–6 times or until you feel your core, arm, and chest muscles starting to tire.

Dynamic Warm-Up

The following dynamic sequence should be completed before beginning each workout. The sequence will only take around 3–4 minutes to complete but is essential for making sure that your body is fully prepared before working out. Don't ever be tempted to skip these exercises because doing so could lead to discomfort and, at worst, injury. If you find yourself with more time to warm up, then go through these exercises a second time, accentuating each move on your second round. The longer that you give yourself to warm up, the better, not only for your body physically but also for you, mentally. Sometimes, after only a short warm-up, going into higher intensity exercise too soon can make your muscles, and your head, give up. Whenever you can, allow yourself more time and enjoy a long, slow warm-up that relaxes your mind. Doing this will remove any feelings of anxiety you may have about the workout. At the same time your muscles can gradually gear-up without feeling any stress or strain. This puts both your mind and body in exactly the right zone to have a really great workout.

Before beginning your dynamic sequence you need to have completed 2–4 minutes of your first workout exercise, as indicated on your workout guidelines. The aim of these initial warm-up minutes is to start your body moving, increasing your body's temperature and blood flow to your muscles, so that your muscles and joints become more receptive to your dynamic moves. These initial exercises must be done at a low intensity and with small ranges of movement so that you don't feel discomfort. Aim to work at a level where your breathing remains normal and where you feel you are exercising, but not so much that you body feels jarred, or stretched, by the activity.

The following is a sequence of exercises that are designed gradually to lengthen muscles and enable your joints to move more freely, preparing your body fully for your fat burner workouts. These exercises take the place of more traditional stretching, often used at the beginning of a workout. As mentioned in the introduction, these dynamic moves are far more effective for warming up, especially when time is limited. By following these exercises you will be able to warm up effectively and in a relatively short space of time.

It is important to try to keep your body moving while you focus on a particular muscle area. The muscle area that you need to be aware of is indicated in each step of the sequence; for example, step 1 works on the front of your shoulder and chest, step 2 on the middle and lower back. Picture this part of your body in your mind's eye to help you increase your focus on this area. Use slow but definite movements, starting small then gradually increasing in size. You should move continuously as you repeat each motion. Avoid any jerky, fast movements and breathe deeply. As you get used to the sequence you should find that you are able to move swiftly and smoothly from one step to the next.

Dynamic Warm-Up

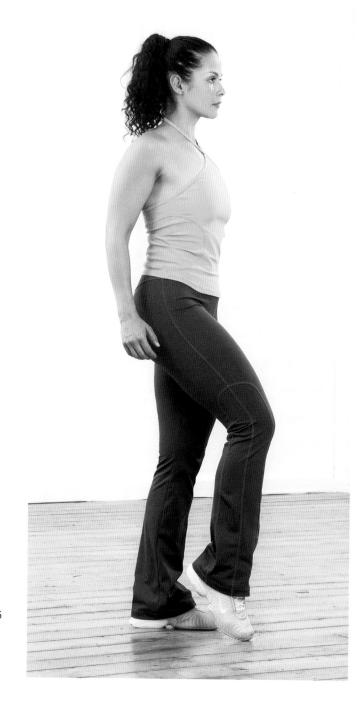

Method

Step 1

- March on the spot and circle your shoulders backward.
- Focus on good postural alignment: midsection in, back tall. Repeat this 10–15 times using large, slow circles. You should aim to feel a lengthening at the front of your shoulders and chest and a loosening through your upper back.

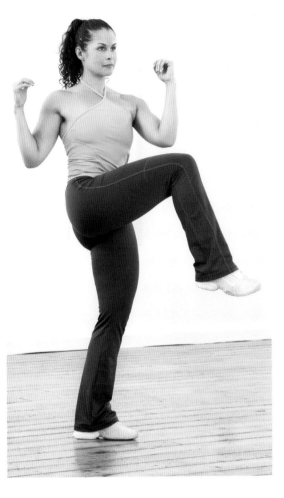

Step 3

- Now, with your feet hip-width apart, take a large step forward with your left foot, bending your left knee so that it comes in line (or remains in line) with your left ankle while keeping your right leg straight, heel just lifting off the ground.
- Your step should be just wide enough to hold your right heel close, but not quite touching, the floor. Your focus when you reach this position should be on a lengthening feeling down the back of your lower right leg.
- Hold your right arm forward and left arm back in a running action.

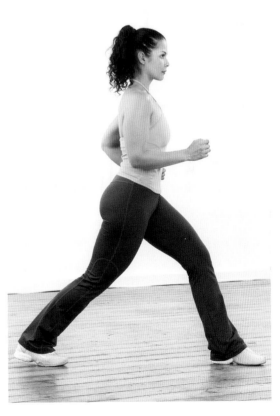

Step 2

- Move on to lifting up your knees alternately.
- At the same time lift the opposite elbow forward and rotate at your waist to mobilize your middle and lower back.
- Keep your back tall at all times and move slowly and carefully through your waist, going only as far as your back feels comfortable.
- Repeat this 10 times on each knee and waist rotation (20 in total).

Dynamic Warm-Up

Step 4

- Keeping your torso lifted in correct postural alignment—stomach in, back tall, shoulders back—bend your right knee to bring your right thigh forward.
- At the same time swing your right arm back and left arm forward.
- Your focus when in this position should be on a lengthening feeling at the top of your right thigh.
- Repeat this action, going back to the position in step 3 and focussing on lengthening the right lower leg by pressing your right heel back toward the floor, then slowly bending your right knee to push your thigh forward, feeling a lengthening down the front of your thigh. Do this 8–10 times.

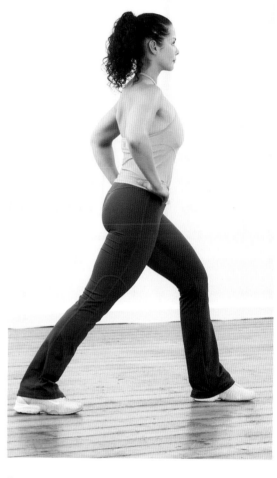

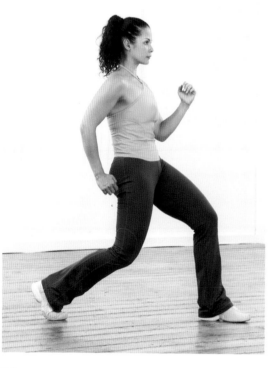

Step 5

- Return your legs to the position in Step 3, bend your right knee, and place your hands on your hips.
- If you have a weak back, as an alternative you may wish to place your hands on your left thigh instead. Be careful, however, not to press down too heavily, as this could cause pressure on your left knee joint.

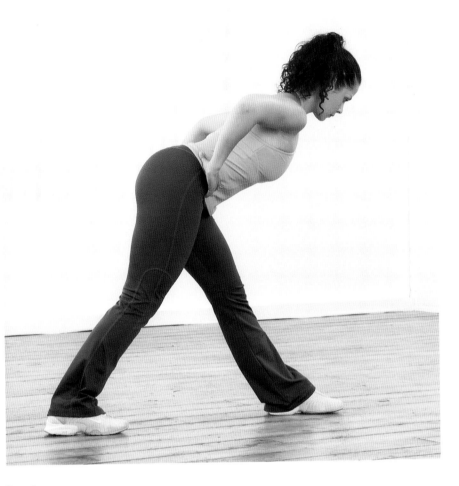

Step 6

- Slowly lean forward with your torso and straighten out your left leg.
- It's really important here to maintain your back's natural curves, so be careful not to round your back.
- Push your butt back slightly and keep connecting to your core, especially your abdominals and pelvic floor muscles.
- As you lean forward you should start to feel a lengthening down the back of your left thigh.
- You need to move more slowly through this movement to ensure your back feels comfortable throughout. Aim to take 4 slow counts to lower enough to feel a stretch.
- Return to step 5 slowly over 4 counts and repeat 4–6 times, gradually increasing the length down the back of your thigh each time.

Finish

- Change legs so that your right leg is in front and your left leg is behind.
- Go back through the sequence from steps 4 to 6, repeating the same action on the opposite side.

Walking and Running

Walking and running are excellent fat burning activities that are easy to take up and can be included as a workout session on their own, or as part of one of your alternative outdoor sessions. If using these as alternatives to your Cardio Circuit sessions, simply aim to run, walk, or do a combination of the two (see below). You need to begin with a warm-up and finish with a cool-down, following the same guidelines as in all your other workouts. It is important, however, to get your running and walking technique right.

Learning to walk before you run

Walking is an ideal activity if you are a beginner or if you suffer from injuries that may make running unsuitable for you. You may be thinking, "Why do I need to be taught how to walk?" While we do successfully learn how to walk as a child, in adulthood we adopt bad habits, from poor posture through to inefficient stride and technique. By adopting the correct form for walking you will maximize the use of your muscles and burn more fat.

Running and Walking Technique

Running and walking are repetitive activities, which, if performed incorrectly, can cause undue stress. This is something that you may not notice in relaxed walking or in a short sprint to catch a train. Using incorrect technique for prolonged periods ,however, leads to a less efficient workout and could cause discomfort in areas such as your back, knees, and hips. Try to memorize the five points on the next pages for when you go out on a walk or run. While on your workout, go through each point, starting from your your heel strike and then working up through your body until you are concentrating on your shoulders and neck. By focussing on your body like this as you go through each point you will not only improve your efficiency but will also find it easier to keep going until your 20 minutes is up.

By following these guidelines on how to run and walk effectively you will reap greater benefits from your fat burning plan.

To begin effective fat burner running, try the following start-up guide. Make sure you warm up by walking for at least 5 minutes first and cool down using the cool-down stretches.

Week 1 Walk briskly for 4 minutes and run for 1, repeat this x 4 to complete 20 minutes

Week 2 Walk briskly for 3 minutes and run for 2, repeat this x 4 to complete 20 minutes

Week 3 Walk briskly for 2 minutes and run for 3, repeat this x 4 to complete 20 minutes

Week 4 Again, walk briskly for 2 minutes and run for 3, repeat this x 4 to complete 20 minutes

Week 5 Walk briskly for 1 minute and run for 4, repeat this x 4 to complete 20 minutes

Week 6 Run continuously for 20 minutes.

Walking and Running

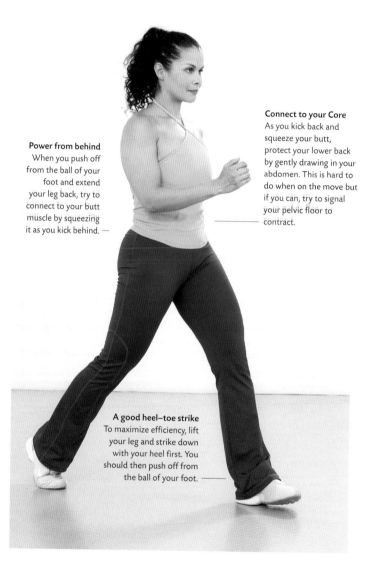

Power from behind
When you push off from the ball of your foot and extend your leg back, try to connect to your butt muscle by squeezing it as you kick behind. —

Connect to your Core
As you kick back and squeeze your butt, protect your lower back by gently drawing in your abdomen. This is hard to do when on the move but if you can, try to signal your pelvic floor to contract.

A good heel–toe strike
To maximize efficiency, lift your leg and strike down with your heel first. You should then push off from the ball of your foot. —

Keeping up your intensity

As you become fitter, you will need to set yourself new challenges. Remember from your intensity guidelines (see page 10) how the exercise should feel: you should be slightly out of breath, breaking into a sweat, heart rate raised, challenged, but able to keep going for at least 20 minutes. If you feel your walking or running is getting easier, increase the intensity by planning a new route to include flights of steps or hills. Try to find a route where within the 20 minutes you get at least four challenges that last at least a minute each. If you can only find one or two suitable hills or steps, work in a circuit, repeating them a second time.

Once you have mastered this your aim should not be to speed up but to try to lengthen your walk or run. This

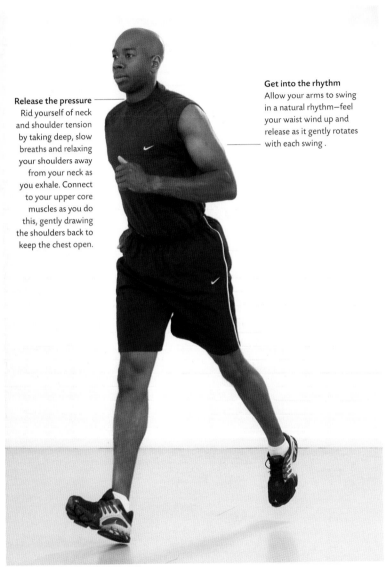

Note

All points shown in the pictures of Kim and Stan refer to both running and walking.

Release the pressure
Rid yourself of neck and shoulder tension by taking deep, slow breaths and relaxing your shoulders away from your neck as you exhale. Connect to your upper core muscles as you do this, gently drawing the shoulders back to keep the chest open.

Get into the rhythm
Allow your arms to swing in a natural rhythm—feel your waist wind up and release as it gently rotates with each swing .

means keeping going at a steady pace. With running this is easier said than done. To help you with this, always start off at a slow jog where you almost feel you could walk faster than you are running. Increase your pace gradually.

Avoiding runner's burnout

Running is a high-impact activity. At some point during your running action both of your feet will lift off the ground at the same time. As you land, this increases the forces that go through your body, which is why many of us find running so uncomfortable.

Running is therefore not always suited to everyone, especially if you are very overweight or have injury concerns. If you follow the above guidelines, however, you may be pleasantly surprised to find that you can learn to run. The effort required to run is a lot higher than that of walking. Running is therefore one of the most effective way to burn calories; but it is only any good as a fat burning activity if you can learn to keep it going for a minimum of 20 minutes.

Fat Burner
Strength Exercises

Traditional strength exercises often tend to focus on one area of the body, with workouts centered on training a particular body part. While this is great for getting to grips with toning or adding strength to certain areas, it doesn't always tackle our main focus—fat. It is often assumed that we can "spot reduce," that is, work on a particular body part and hey presto, a once droopy butt becomesd pert and fat free. While I wish this was true, the facts are as follows:

• Muscle lies underneath fat, so if you want to see a toned body part you need to get rid of the fat that lies over the top.

• Doing targeted exercises, while working muscles effectively, will not remove the fat specifically from that area.

• To remove fat you need to do exercises that generate enough energy expenditure to metabolize fat from the whole body. This involves doing large, whole body movements which work you up into a sweat and, through sustained periods of energy transfer, cause you to burn fat.

• Some areas will lose fat more easily than others. Abdominal fat, for example, is easier to metabolize than hip and thigh fat. You may therefore find it easier to lose fat around your abdomen than your hips and thighs.

Persevere nevertheless, as you will lose fat over all areas if you stick to regular training and healthy eating.

• We are what we are! Our body shape is largely dictated by genetics and while we can increase muscle size and reduce fat levels to help balance things out, your overall shape, for example, small shoulders with big hips, or a thick waist with stick legs, will tend to remain more or less the same.

• The good news is, however, that through exercise you can make your shape dramatically better, changing, for example, from a large pear to a small juicy one, with sculpted shoulders and a very fashionable butt (think Beyonce or J-Lo!)

The following exercises, therefore, are designed to incorporate whole body movements, ensuring that you maximize muscle usage and burn fat while also strengthening and toning all areas of the body. Work with slow, controlled movements and remember to activate your core muscles, especially when you exert most pressure, that is, as you lift, press, push, or pull. Always breathe out at this point and keep your mind on the exercise focus. Each exercise has a tougher next step, given in the Hints & Tips box. You should aim to follow this when you have been doing the exercises for at least four weeks and feel that you need an extra challenge.

Strength–Beginners

squat and row

Aim: To work the legs, buttocks, and core muscles in a holding position while using your front arm (Bicep), back, and waist muscles to pull a resistance band.

Focus: Concentrate on your middle area, from your waist at the front (Obliques), to underneath your shoulder blade (Latissimus Dorsi and Lower Trapezius).

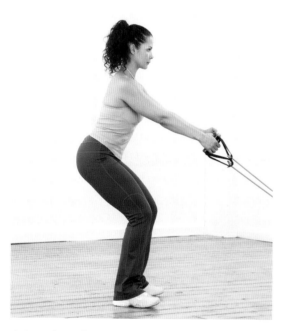
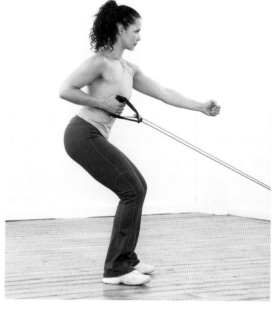

Method

- Position your band around a fixed bed leg or low hook/pole.
- Take hold of both handles in your right hand and stand far away enough from the support to generate mild tension in the band.
- Sit back into a half-squat position, paying attention to your back posture.
- Connect to your core and hold both arms out in front, while keeping your shoulders back and down.
- Take a breath in and, as you breathe out, pull with your right arm, focussing on pulling from your back and waist. Your left arm should naturally come forward as your waist slightly rotates.
- Finish with your elbow behind and a strong contraction under your shoulder blades and through your waist.

Hints & Tips

- Check in a mirror to ensure that you are holding your back in its natural curves.
- Be careful not to allow the elbow to lift—focus on drawing down as you pull back.
- When pulling from the right, pull back with your waist muscles on the left side to keep your hips square to the front. Do the opposite when pulling from the left.
- To progress, swap to your harder band and use a rhythm of pulling for 2 counts, releasing for 4.

- Slowly release the band and repeat 15–20 times or until the muscles in your back and waist start to tire. Change sides.

seated ball press

Aim: To hold a good seated posture while working the main muscles of the chest and the Tricep muscle on the back of your arm.

Focus: Concentrate on using your core and chest muscles (Pectoralis Major), as you press forward with your arms (Triceps).

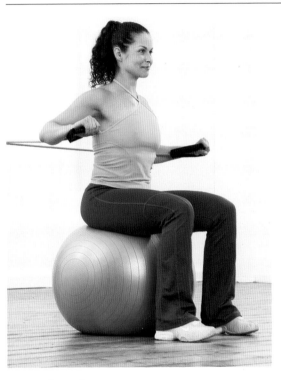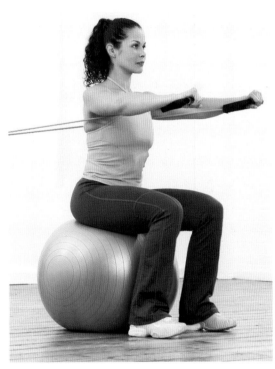

Method

- Fix the middle of your lighter weight band to a hook or handle, level with your (sitting) chest height.
- Sit tall on your ball and take a hold of each handle, making sure the band goes underneath your arms.
- Position your elbows low and behind you, so that your hands come back in line with your chest. There should be mild tension in the band in this position.
- Connect to your core, take a breath in and, checking that your shoulders stay back and down, press slowly through with both arms as you breathe out.
- Fully extend the arms without allowing your shoulders to come forward and without closing out at your elbow joint.
- Keeping your core well connected, slowly release the band back to the starting point.
- Repeat the exercise 15–20 times or until the muscles in your chest and arms start to tire .

Hints & Tips

- Concentrate on pushing through the chest: muscles first, then the arms.
- Help to keep your shoulders low by drawing the back of your neck into a lengthened position and pulling back with your chin to keep your nose pointing forward.
- To progress, swap to your harder band and use a rhythm of pulling for 2 counts and releasing slowly for 4 counts.

seated rotate and lift

Aim: To work the waist and shoulder muscles (the Deltoids) with maximum energy.
Focus: Concentrate on using all the muscles of your trunk and arms to keep your back tall and pull the band around. You should feel fatigued in the muscle at the top of your arm.

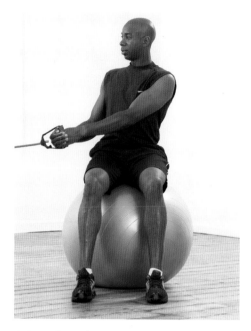

Hints & Tips

- Imagine you are rotating around a vertical column that is your spine.
- Pull from your abdominals and waist first, then bring the arms around.
- Ensure that your shoulders don't lift into your neck. Keep focussing on core muscles to keep the shoulders back and down.
- To progress, swap to your harder band and pull for 2 counts, releasing slowly for 4 counts.

- Finish with your arms lifted to the left side, left elbow bent and just below shoulder height, and right arm extended in front.
- Slowly release back to the start and repeat 15–20 times or until your arms and shoulders start to tire. Change sides.

Method

- Using your lighter band, position one end of the band around a fixed bed leg or low hook/pole.
- With your right side nearest the band, sit on the ball and hold onto the handle with both hands, left hand over the top of your right.
- Your right arm should be bent to your side, left, nearly straight in front, creating a mild tension in the band.
- Connect to your core, take a breath in and as you breathe out start to pull through your waist and arms.

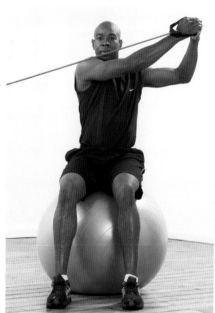

wide squat

Aim: To establish correct lifting and lowering techniques while working your legs, buttocks and inner thigh muscles.
Focus: Maintain correct back posture, working your weight back into your heels and squeezing through your main buttock muscle (Gluteus Maximus) to lift.

Method

- Hold onto on to one of your heavier dumbbells (8 lb.) at one end.
- Stand with your feet wider than hip-width, feet turned out at 45 degrees.
- Check your posture by using a mirror and connect to your core.
- Take a breath and as you breathe out, lower back into a squat position, weight into your heels, as if sitting back onto a chair.

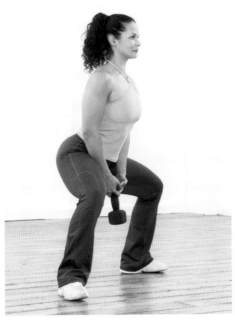

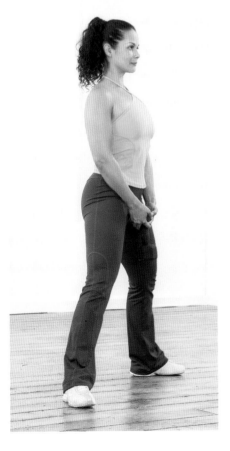

- Lower to a point just above 90 degrees at the knee joint.
- Hold this position for a few seconds and recheck your posture: your knees should be behind your toes.
- Take another breath and, as you breathe out, reconnect to your core and lift, pushing your weight through your heels and using your butt.

Hints & Tips

- Be careful when picking up heavy weights—use the squat to lift, keeping your back tall.
- Stand sideways on to a mirror and keep checking your back to ensure it maintains its natural curves.
- To progress, increase your weight and hold the squat for 6–10 counts before lifting back up.

single lat pulldown

Aim: To maintain core stability while working the back and opening the chest muscles.
Focus: Concentrate on your abdominal core muscles while squeezing into the back muscles (Latissimus Dorsi) as your elbow draws into your ribs.

Method

- Sit tall on the ball and, using your lighter weight band, double it over, holding both handles with your right hand and the loop end with your left.
- Place the band behind your head elbows at 90 degrees, shoulders drawn back and down. The band should maintain mild tension.
- Connect to your core and, as you breathe out, pull the right side of the band down, anchoring the loop end by keeping your left arm still.

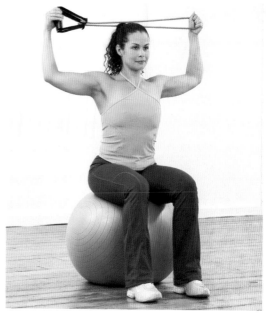

- Squeeze down on your back muscles as you bring your elbow into your side.
- Slowly release the band and repeat 15–20 times or until you feel your back muscles starting to tire. Change sides.

Hints & Tips

- It is important to lock hold of your core abdominal muscles to prevent your lower back from over-arching.
- Aim to maximize the length in your chest by keeping your head up tall and really squeezing your shoulders blades together.
- To progress, swap to using your harder band and for an extra challenge, try taking one foot off the floor. This will increase the work on your core muscles. Make sure you keep your back tall and hips level.

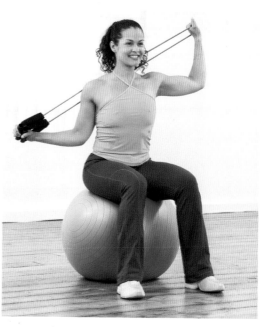

standing tricep extension

Aim: To hold good core posture while strengthening and toning the back of your arm.

Focus: The back arm muscle (Triceps), maximizing the control of your abdominal and pelvic floor muscles.

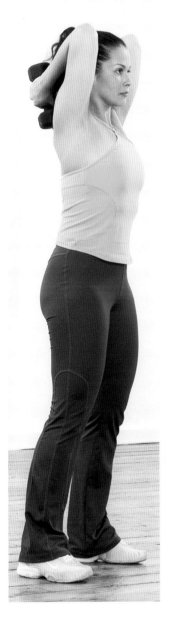

Method

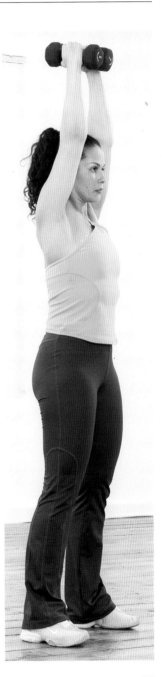

- Stand with your feet hip-width apart.
- Using 2–4 lb. dumbbells, hold a weight in each hand and raise them up and over your head.
- Aim to have your upper arm by your ears and your forearm and weights dropped low behind your back.
- Work hard, pulling in your abdominals and pelvic floor muscles to prevent your lower back from overarching.
- Take a breath and as you breathe out, carefully extend both arms up toward the ceiling, focussing on squeezing your Tricep muscle.
- Slowly lower the forearm and repeat 15–20 times or until your arms begin to tire.

Hints & Tips

- If you have tight shoulders and find it difficult to get your arms behind your head, work one arm at a time, keeping the working arm in place by supporting it with your free hand.
- Straighten your arms without closing out at the elbow joint.
- Increase your weight for an extra challenge and/or try to balance on one leg. You will have to really concentrate on your core muscles to help you balance. Change legs halfway through.

forward lunges

Aim: To strengthen and tone the legs and buttock muscles while maintaining core control.
Focus: Maximize the use of your butt muscle (Gluteus Maximus) by talking yourself through the correct heel-toe-heel action and concentrating on lifting through your Glutes.

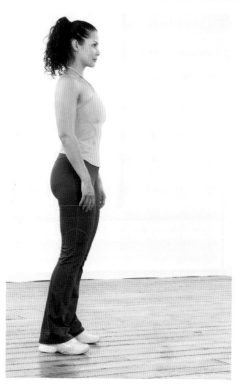

Method

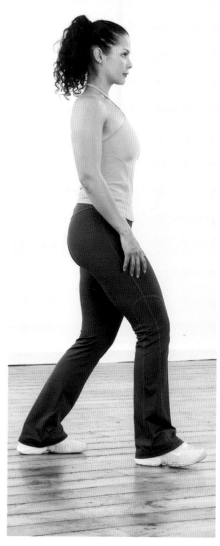

- Stand with your feet hip-width apart and check your posture.
- Connect to your core and take a small step forward with your right foot
- Strike down with your heel, roll onto the ball of your foot, then push back from your heel to the start position. Practice these small steps a few times to get used to the heel-toe-heel technique.
- Now take a larger step, with your right leg stepped out in front.
- Hold this position and with your weight into your right heel, slowly bend at the knees to reach a lunge position, no lower than 90 degrees at each knee.

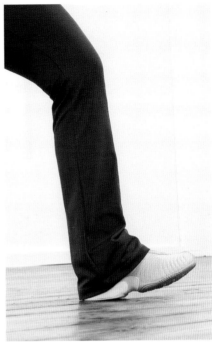

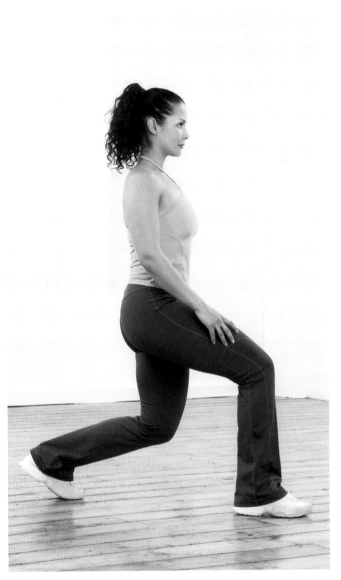

- Take a breath and as you breathe out slowly push back up with your weight into your right heel.
- Focus on using your buttock muscles to pull back to the start.
- Repeat 20–30 alternating lunges (10–15 on each leg).

Hints & Tips

- Avoid pushing your body weight forward by aiming to keep your spine vertical at all times.
- Check that your front knee stays behind your toes in the lunged position.
- To progress, hold 5–8 lb. dumbbells to make the exercise harder. Make sure that the weights do not pull your shoulders forward by focussing on your shoulder and back core muscles.

49

towel ab curl

Aim: To strengthen and tone the outer Abdominals while also maintaining core control.
Focus: Concentrate on a contraction between the bottom of the ribs and the navel, while aiming to keep the lower abdomen hollowed as you lift.

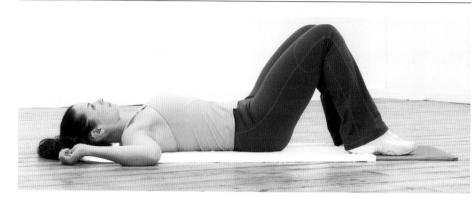

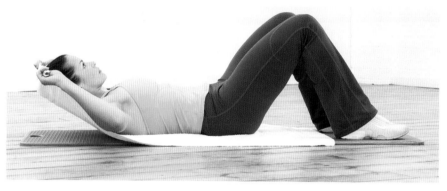

Method

- Lie on the floor on your towel, head close to the top of the towel, feet hip-width apart.
- Make sure you have a little hollow in your lower back, butt on the floor.
- Take a hold of each top corner of the towel with each hand and focus on drawing in and down with your core back and shoulder muscles.
- Take a breath in and, as you breathe out, lift your head neck, shoulders, arms, and towel off the floor.
- Keep your head back into your towel as you lift, focus on bringing your rib cage in toward your navel.
- At the same time, aim to keep your lower back in its natural small arch, using your core abdominal muscles to hollow your abdomen and keep your lower back in place.

- Lower your back toward the floor without quite touching your head to the ground.
- Repeat 15–20 times or until your abs start to tire.

Hints & Tips

- To prevent neck strain, draw your chin back into your neck without looking down and relax your head back into the towel.
- To prevent strain in your shoulders and arms, focus on your shoulder and back core muscles, pulling them down to support the upper body.
- To progress, place your lightest dumbbells in each hand and grip onto the towel as before.

foot lifts

Aim: To strengthen the lower section of your abdominals and help to flatten your stomach.

Focus: Concentrate on your pelvic floor and deep abdominals, using them to keep your pelvis still as you lift each foot.

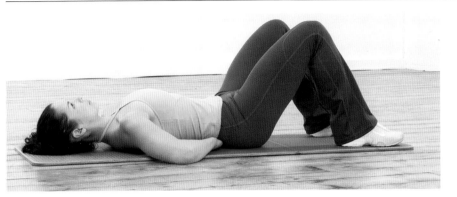

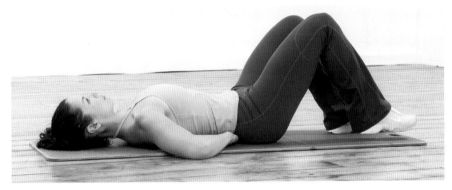

Method

- Lie on your back, feet hip-width apart and knees in line with your hips.
- Make sure you have a small arch in your lower back, butt relaxed on the floor.
- Draw your shoulders down, away from your neck, and connect gently to your core.
- Take a deep slow breath and as you breathe out, carefully lift your right foot off the floor.
- As you lift your foot, draw in your core abdomen and PF muscles as much as you can to prevent your hips from moving or your stomach from bulging.
- Carefully lower your foot so that the pelvis does not shift as you lower.
- Make sure your back has maintained its natural small curve, checking with your fingers.

Hints & Tips

- To help flatten the stomach its important not to allow it to bulge out. If you feel this is happening, lift your heel, not the whole foot.
- To progress, lift one foot as before, then tilt your pelvis to press your lower back into your fingers. Making sure your abdomen stays drawn in, take another breath and as you exhale, lift your second foot so that both are off the floor. Return both feet and spine back to the start. Repeat 6–10 times.

- Repeat lifting with your left foot then continue lifting right then left 6 to 10 times each or until you feel you can't hold your pelvis in the correct position.

51

seated outward rotation

Aim: To work the back (Rhomboids and lower Trapezius) and shoulder (Deltoid) muscles while also lengthening the chest (Pectoralis Major), improving posture and core strength. Focus: Keep your shoulders back and down throughout. You should feel the back muscles between your shoulder blades working all the time. Keep your elbows close to your ribs through the first two stages and, as you lift, focus on a feeling in your outer shoulder area.

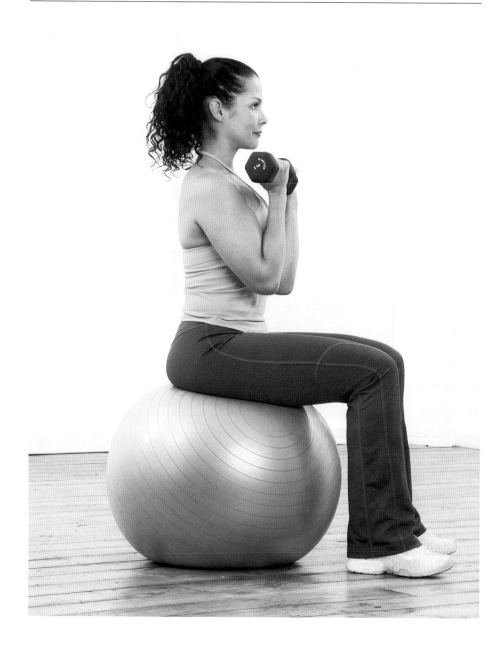

Method

- Sit tall on your ball, feet hip-width apart, core muscles connected.
- Using 2 lb. dumbbells, hold a weight in each hand and position your arms, bent in front of your chest with thumbs turned out, palms to chest.
- Keep them close to your body by focussing on drawing your shoulders back and down.

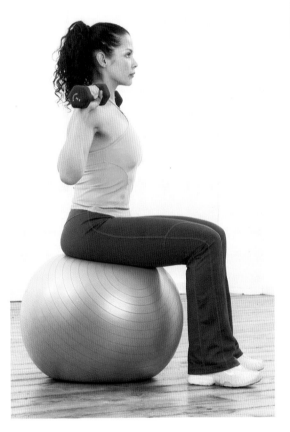

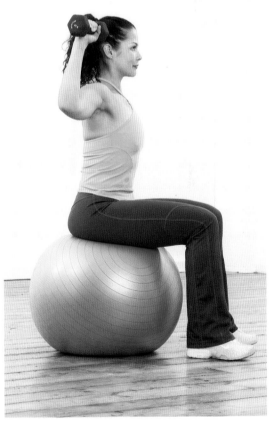

- Working hard to keep your elbows close to your side, take a breath and as you breathe out, work your arms around to the side until your elbow is level with your shoulder.
- Aim to work really hard at squeezing the muscles between your shoulder blades.
- Take another breath and as you breathe out, carefully lift your elbow up to shoulder height.
- Keep your shoulder blades squeezed in and down as you lift, lower and repeat 10–15 times.

single leg glute lift

Aim: To work your large buttock muscle (Gluteus Maximus) and back of your thigh.

Focus: Concentrate mainly on squeezing your Gluteus Maximus while also being aware of your posture on the bench.

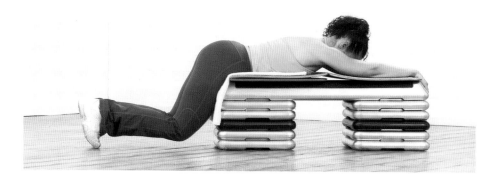

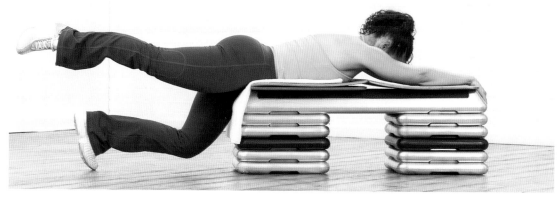

Method

- Stack your step bench high enough for you to lie on without your knees touching the floor. You could use a bed or suitably stable low table instead.
- Lie on the bench with your hips coming off the end.
- Hold on to the end of the bench with your hands and draw your shoulders back and down.
- Take a breath and as you breathe out, lift your right foot off the floor.
- Work hard on your core muscles here to hold you still on the step.
- Slowly and carefully extend your right leg out, keeping your pelvis down on the bench.
- As your leg extends and lifts, squeeze your butt muscle and be careful not to push into your lower back.

Hints & Tips

- Be careful not to lift too high. Once you have reached hip height, pull your abs in to protect your back and focus on extending your leg away, rather than up.
- Make sure that your pelvis is comfortable on the bench—you can do this by placing a mat or a folded towel under your torso and over the end of the bench.
- To progress, take both feet off the floor and work harder on your core muscles to hold you on the bench. Lift as before.

- Slowly lower and repeat leg 15–20 times or until you feel your butt muscle start to tire. Change legs.

Strength–Advanced

single leg squat and row

Aim: To work the legs, butt, and core muscles as you balance on one leg, while using your front arm (Bicep), back, and waist muscles to pull the band.

Focus: Concentrate on your middle area, from your waist at the front (Obliques), to underneath your shoulder blade (Latissimus Dorsi and Lower Trapezius).

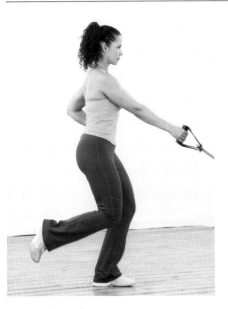 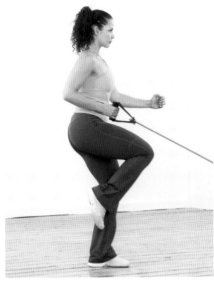

Method

- Position your band around a fixed bed leg or low hook or pole.
- Take hold of both handles in your right hand and stand far away enough from the support to generate mild tension in the band.
- Stand on your left leg and sit back slightly to bend your knee.
- Connect to your core and hold both arms out in front, while keeping your shoulders back and down.
- Take a breath in and as you breathe out, start to pull with your right arm, focussing on pulling from your back and waist. Your left arm and right knee should naturally come forward as your waist slightly rotates.
- At the same time allow your left leg to straighten.
- Finish with your elbow behind you and a strong contraction under your shoulder blades and through your waist.

- Slowly release the band and lower back into your half squat position. Repeat 15–20 times or until the muscles in your back, waist, and legs start to tire. Change sides.

Hints & Tips

- Be careful not to allow the elbow to lift—focus on drawing down as you pull back.
- When pulling from the right, pull back with your waist muscles on the left side to keep your hips square to the front. Do the opposite when pulling from the left.
- To progress, swap to your harder band and use a rhythm of pulling for 2 counts and releasing slowly for 4 counts.

lying ball press

Aim: To stabilize on the ball using your buttocks (Gluteus Maximus) and core abdominal muscles while opening out and strengthening the chest.

Focus: Concentrate on keeping your hips up, using your core abdominals and glutes.

Method

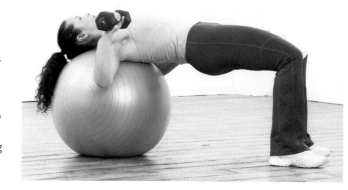

- Choose one medium dumbbell and sit on the ball holding the weight centrally across your chest
- Slowly and carefully lower yourself into a lying position by walking your legs forward and lower your back towards the ball. Draw in with your abdominals as you lower.
- Once your back is on the ball, keep walking your feet forward until your shoulders are resting on the middle apex of the ball.
- Place the weight into your right hand and draw your right elbow down along the side of the ball, knuckles facing up to bring the weight in line with your chest.
- Push your hips up until your thighs are parallel with your pelvis, being careful not to over-arch your back. Keep your knees and feet hip-width apart. Draw in your abdominals and squeeze your buttocks.
- Take a breath in and, as you breathe out press your right arm up toward the ceiling, bringing the weight over your chest.
- Keeping your core, well connected, hips lifted, slowly release the weight back to the start position
- Repeat the exercise 15–20 times or until the muscles in your chest and arm start to tire. Change sides.

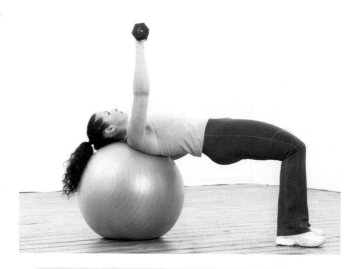

Hints & Tips

- Concentrate on pushing through the chest muscles first, then the arms.
- To help keep your hips and legs in the right position, place a rolled up towel between your knees.
- To progress, increase the weight of your dumbbell and use a rhythm of pushing for two counts and lowering slowly for 4 counts.

squat, rotate, and lift

Aim: To work the legs, buttock, waist, and shoulder muscles (Deltoids) with maximum energy.

Focus: Concentrate on using all the muscles of your trunk, buttocks, and arms to keep your back tall and pull the band around. Aim to feel fatigued in the muscle at the top of your arm, the Deltoid.

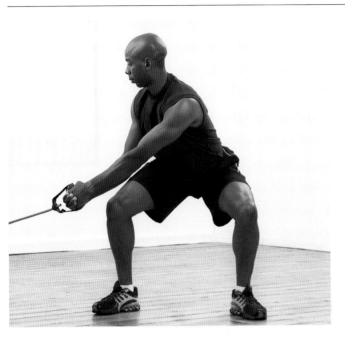

Method

- Using a lighter band, position one handle around a fixed bed leg or low hook or pole.
- With your right side nearest the band, hold the handle with both hands.
- Take your legs into a wide squat position, feet turned out at 45 degrees and lower into a squat, with your arms to your right side. Position yourself to create a mild tension in the band.
- Connect to your core, paying particular attention to keep the shoulders back and chest lifted.
- Take a breath in and as you breathe out start to lift out of the squat and pull the band up and around to the left.
- Start to allow the right leg to pivot, adding power to the movement as you rotate around to the left-hand side.
- Finish with your arms lifted to the left side and your right leg pivoted around to the left on the ball of you foot.
- Slowly release back to the start and repeat 15–20 times or until your arms and shoulders start to tire. Change sides.

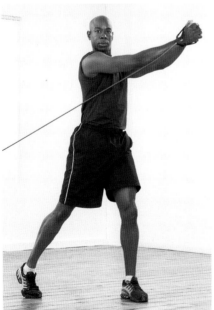

Hints & Tips

- Imagine you are rotating around a vertical column, that is, your spine.
- As you lift through your legs, pull from your abdominals and waist first, then bring the arms around.
- Be careful that your shoulders don't lift into your neck. Keep focussing on core muscles to keep the shoulders back and down, back tall.
- To progress, swap to a harder band, pulling for 2 counts and releasing slowly for 4 counts.

lunge back and lift

Aim: To establish correct lifting and lowering techniques while working your legs (hamstrings and Quadriceps), butt (Gluteus Maximus), shoulder (Deltoids), and arms.

Focus: Concentrate on maintaining the correct back posture, holding your weight close to your chest as you lunge, maximizing the control of your upper core muscles.

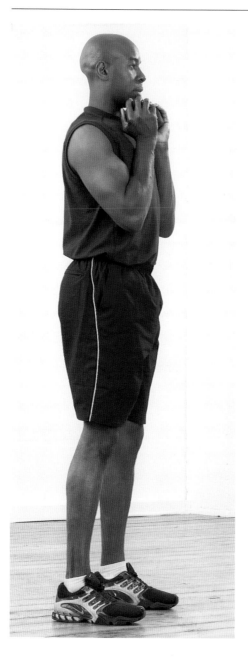

Method

- Using correct lifting technique, as in your Posture Squat (see Core Exercises, page 26), pick up one of your heavier dumbbells (10–15 lb./4.5–7 kg) and hold as shown with one hand on each end.
- Stand with your feet hip-width apart and connect to all your core muscles.
- Take a breath and as you breathe out, step back with your right leg into a back lunge position with your knees at about a 90-degree angle.)
- Lift back up by pushing through your left heel. (Continued on page 60.)

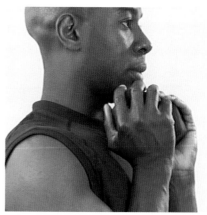

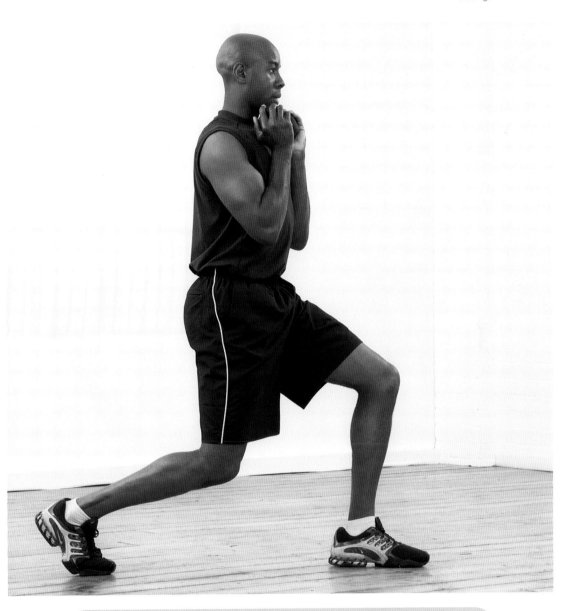

Hints & Tips

- If you find it difficult to balance on one leg, start by keeping the ball of your right foot on the ground as you press up with your arms.
- Makes sure your torso stays vertical as you lower into the lunge and that your front knee stays behind your toes.
- To progress, increase the weight and aim to hold your balance on one leg for longer by doing two arm lifts for every one lunge.

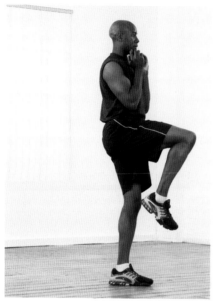

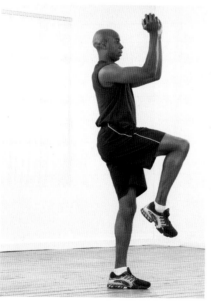

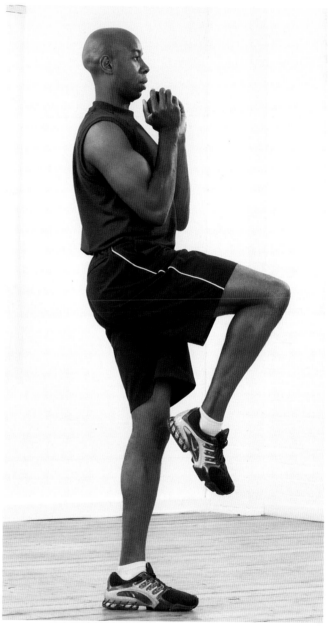

- As you lift back up, aim to keep your right foot off the floor.
- When your left leg is near to an extended position, take another breath and, as you breathe out, reconnect to your core and lift the weight up to bring your elbows to shoulder height, keeping your shoulders down and away from your neck.
- Lower, aiming to keep your right foot off the ground. Repeat with the right leg 6–8 times, then change legs.

straight arm pull down

Aim: To maintain core stability in a squat position while working the back (Latissimus Dorsi) muscles.

Focus: Concentrate on your abdominal core muscles while squeezing into the back muscles as your elbow draws into your ribs.

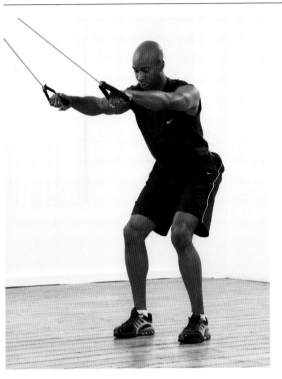
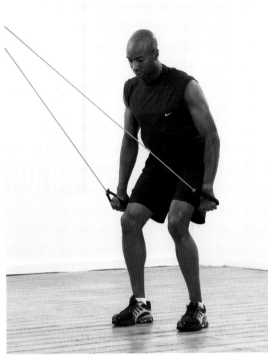

Method

- Attach your easier band to a high hook or pole. If your band is not long enough to give you the correct movement, you may need to use both bands, attaching your harder one to the high fixed position and then looping your easier band through its handles.
- Hold onto the handles of your easier band and half-squat back so that the band is under mild tension.
- With your arms extended up and in front, connect to your core and, as you breathe out, pull both handles down together.
- Squeeze down on your back muscles as you bring your elbows into your side.
- Hold and recheck your posture before slowly releasing the band back to the start.
- Repeat 15–20 times or until you feel your back muscles starting to tire.

Hints & Tips

- Keep your shoulders down, even when your arms are in the raised start position
- Your elbows can be slightly soft, but aim to keep the arm in a fixed position as you draw down.
- To help feel the Latissimus Dorsi muscles working, draw your elbows closer into the side of your body, removing any space between your arm and side at the finish point.
- To progress, swap to using a harder band and, for an extra challenge, try taking one foot off the floor. This will work your core muscles intensely and increase your calorie expenditure. Make sure you keep your back tall and hips level.

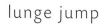
lunge jump

Aim: To challenge the legs (calves, hamstrings, and Quadriceps) and buttocks (Gluteus Maximus), using a powerful movement that increases muscle speed.

Focus: Focus on using your legs as shock absorbers, bending at the knee joint while keeping your torso lifted. Increase the power by pushing up through your buttocks.

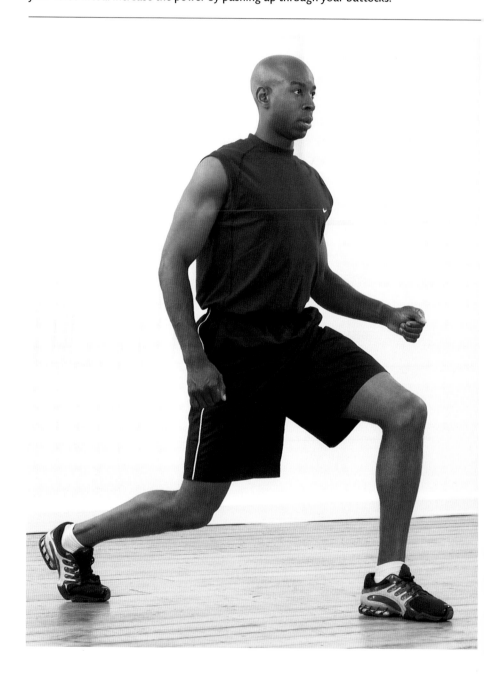

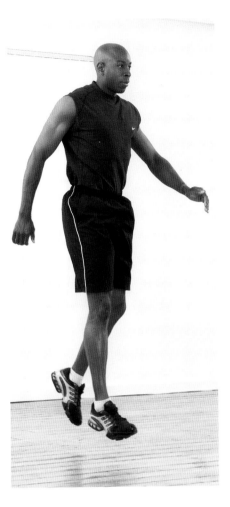

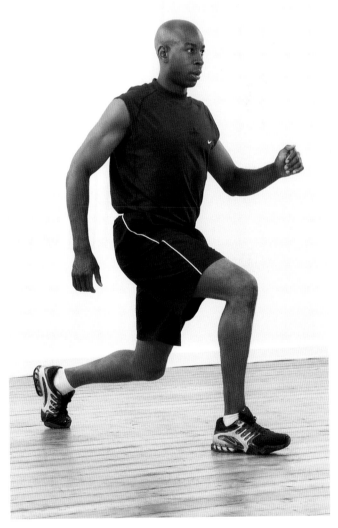

Method

- Start with your feet hip-width apart. Step back with your right leg onto the ball of your foot, feet kept at hip-width.
- Take a breath and as you exhale, connect to your core and drop down slowly into a lunge.
- You should have no more than a 90-degree bend at the front knee joint and with your weight distributed between the left heel and ball of your right foot.
- Quickly lift and jump, pushing through the front heel to switch legs, bringing your right leg to the front. (Continued page 64.)

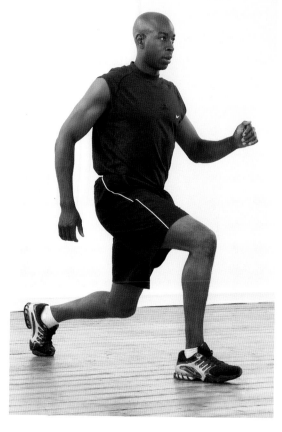

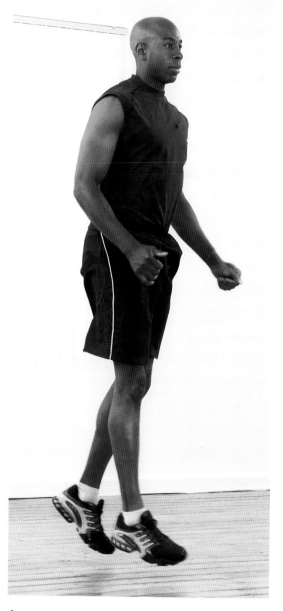

- Immediately jump and switch two more times, so that your right leg finishes in front and your left behind.
- Slowly lower and repeat the process, jumping and switching the legs three times before slowly lowering again to repeat.
- Keep doing this 4–12 times on each side, or until your legs start to tire.

Hints & Tips

- Help to control your balance by thinking about using your core, especially as you land.
- Work in front of a mirror. Check that your knees don't twist out to the side or fall inward as you lower from a jump. Your front knee should not go over your toe as you lower.
- To progress, place your front foot on a step 4–12 inches high and back foot onto the floor as before. Repeat, jumping higher each time.

lying ball tricep extension

Aim: To work the whole body by stabilizing on the ball, while targeting the back of your arm.

Focus: Concentrate on keeping your hips up by squeezing your buttocks and holding your core, while straightening the arm to work the Tricep.

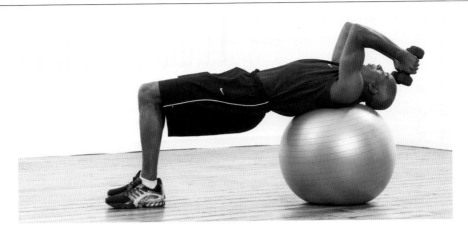

Method

- Hold a light dumbbell in each hand and sit on the ball, holding the weights centrally across your chest.
- Slowly and carefully lower yourself into a lying position by walking your legs forward and lowering your back toward the ball. Draw in with your abdominals as you lower.
- Once your back is on the ball, keep walking your feet forward until your shoulders are resting on the middle apex of the ball.
- Push your hips up until your thighs are parallel with your pelvis, being careful not to over-arch your back. Keep your knees and feet hip-width apart. Squeeze your buttocks and connect to your core.
- Take your arms up until your elbows are vertically aligned with your shoulders and forearms are relaxed behind your head.
- Take a breath in and, as you breathe out, extend your arm up to the ceiling.
- Keeping your core well connected and hips lifted, slowly release the weight back to your start position
- Repeat the movement 15–20 times or until the muscles in the back of your arm begin to tire.

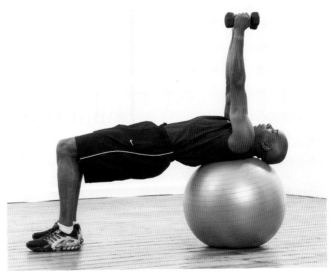

Hints & Tips

- You may find that one arm tires before the other. Rest both arms then take your stronger arm back into position and continue to work it. Now swap to your weaker arm, ensuring that both do the same number of repetitions.
- To progress, increase the weight and/or take your arms further back so that your upper arm is in line with your ears.

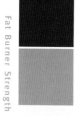

ab curl on the ball

Aim: To strengthen and tone the outer abdominal muscle while also maintaining core control.

Focus: Concentrate on a contraction between the bottom of your ribs and your navel while aiming to keep your lower abdomen hollowed and hips up as you lift.

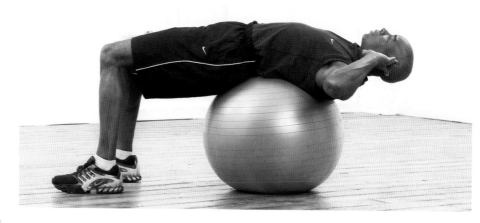

Method

- Sit on the ball and carefully lower yourself into a lying position by walking your legs forward and lowering your back toward the ball. Draw in with your abdominals as you lower.
- Once your back is on the ball, walk your feet backward to bring your head, neck, and shoulders off the ball.
- Take your hands back by the side of your head, draw your chin in and keep the back of your neck long.
- Push your hips up until your thighs are parallel with your pelvis, being careful not to over-arch your back. Keep your knees and feet hip-width apart. Squeeze your buttocks and connect to your core.
- Keeping your head back by your hands, lift, focussing on bringing your rib cage in towards your navel.
- At the same time aim to keep your hips lifted and abdomen flat by using your backside and deep core abdominal muscles.
- Lower back towards the ball and repeat 15–20 times or until your abs start to tire.

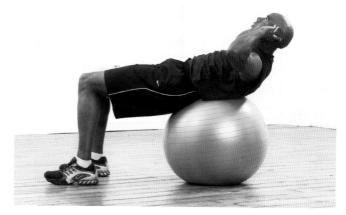

Hints & Tips

- To prevent neck strain and make the exercise slightly easier, rest your head in your hands by interlocking your fingers behind your head.
- Be careful not to push your head and neck forward. Create a double chin to keep your head back in the right position and aim to lift from your ribs to your navel, rather than pulling your head and neck forward.
- To progress, place your lightest dumbbells in each hand and hold with your hands by the side of your head.

double leg glute lifts

Aim: To work your large buttock muscle (Gluteus Maximus) and back of your thigh.
Focus: Concentrate mainly on squeezing your buttocks while also being aware of your posture on the bench.

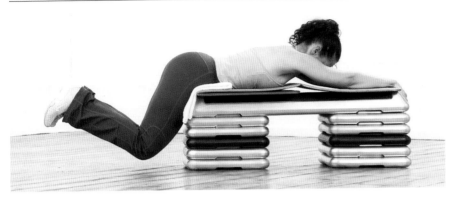

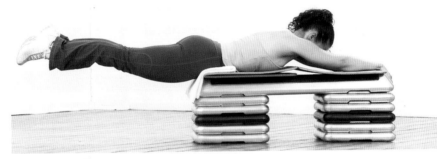

Method

- Stack your step bench up high enough for you to lie on it without your knees touching the floor, or use a bed or a stable low table instead.
- Lie on to the bench with your hips coming off the end.
- Hold on to the end of the bench with your hands, draw your shoulders back and down, and connect to both your upper and lower core muscles.
- Take a breath and as you exhale, lift both legs.
- Work hard on your core muscles to hold you still on the step.
- Slowly and carefully extend both legs, keeping your pelvis down on the bench.
- As your legs extend and lift, squeeze your buttocks and be careful not to push into your lower back.
- Slowly lower and repeat 15–20 times or until you feel your buttocks start to tire.

Hints & Tips

- Be careful not to lift too high. Once you have reached hip height, pull your stomach in to protect your back and focus on extending your leg away rather than up.
- Make sure your pelvis is comfortable on the bench by using a mat and/or a folded towel placed under your torso and over the end of your bench.
- To progress, as you extend your legs, bring your heels and thighs together and rotate out at the hip joint to feel an extra squeeze in your buttocks. Lower and repeat 15–20 times. On the last movement hold your top position for 6–10 counts.

knee drops on step

Aim: To strengthen the lower section of your abdominals and help to flatten your stomach.
Focus: Concentrate on your pelvic floor and deep abdominals, using them to keep your pelvis still as you lift each foot.

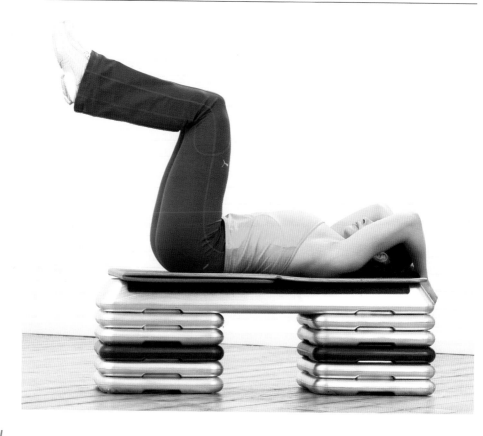

Method

- Lie back on a step bench 10–16 inches high, bringing your knees into your chest.
- Now, lower knees to bring them in line with your hips for a 90-degree angle at your hip joint.
- Start with your pelvis tilted so that you lose the hollow in your lower back. Use your abdominals to draw your pelvis in. Maintain this pressed in position throughout the move.
- Take a breath and, as you exhale, draw in through your abdominals and start to lower one foot toward the floor.

Hints & Tips

- To really help flatten your stomach its important not to allow your abdomen to bulge out as you lower a leg. If you feel this is happening, switch to the Foot Lift exercise in the beginner program and gradually build up to this exercise.
- To progress, begin to lower your foot farther, ensuring that your stomach stays hollowed and the small of your back is pressed to the bench.

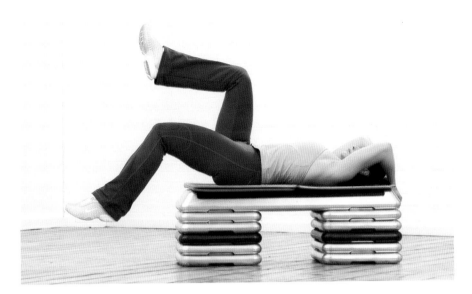

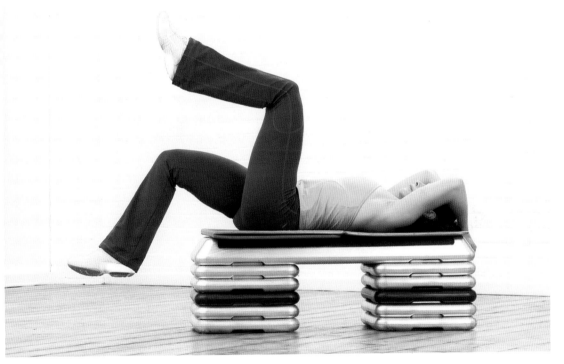

- Lower a short distance at first, making sure that your lower back does not move.
- Bring the knee back to the start and repeat using the other leg.
- Repeat 8–12 times on each leg or until you feel you cannot hold your abdominals in any more.

Cardio Circuit Exercises

The following exercises are designed to improve your cardiovascular (heart and lung) fitness. In addition, they will burn a relatively higher number of calories compared with some of the other exercises, to help with fat loss. You will also find exercises that have been developed to work at slightly higher intensities—this is indicated at the beginning of each exercise description. These exercises appear in the interval-style workouts.

Getting the right intensity for all these exercises is a key factor when it comes to burning the optimum number of calories for each workout. Go back and reread the first section of this book to help you get this right.

For every 20 minutes of a cardio circuit or equivalent workout, for example, you can expect to burn around 2.5–4 calories per 2 lb. of body weight. If you are around 154 lbs and do the equivalent of 2 x 20 minute cardio circuit workouts per week, then through these alone you can burn around 22,682 additional calories in a year!

With interval workouts you can burn even more calories, although the main objective of your interval style workouts is to boost your fitness levels. This, along with your strength exercises, will ultimately help to speed up your metabolism, causing you to burn even more calories.

To reap the full benefit, you need to perform consistently. As well as looking at the intensity guidelines in section one, please bear in mind the following points to keep you on the right track:

• Make sure that you feel able to continue for the time specified for an exercise. Each exercise should feel challenging but achievable.

• Your movement in these exercises will be quicker than in your fat burner strength exercises. You should aim to breathe continuously throughout and try to establish a rhythm to keep you moving at a regular pace.

• Getting the pattern of movement and technique correct is much more important than trying to "go for it" right at the start. To help with this, always begin slowly and gradually build up your speed to an appropriate intensity when you feel you have fully mastered the movement.

• Progressing through the workouts and giving yourself new goals every few weeks is vital to ensure that you continue to burn fat. After every 2–4 weeks you should start to feel the exercises becoming a little easier, and then you can increase intensity, either by carefully increasing your speed or using the harder version of the exercise as provided.

Cardio Circuit–Beginners

step ups

Aim: To build up your heart rate at the beginning of a workout by using the main muscles in the legs and buttocks.

Focus: Concentrate on correct posture and lifting up through your buttocks as you push through your heel and stand tall on the step.

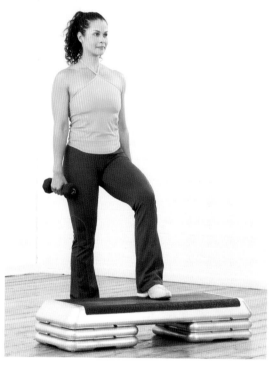 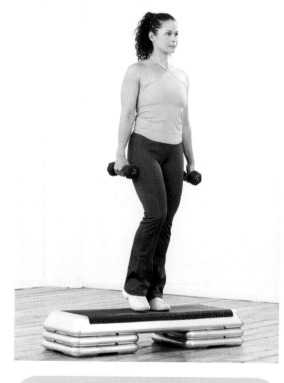

Method

- Use a step 8–10 inches in height. Start without weights if they take you too quickly into your intensity zone.
- Stand within your foot's distance from the step.
- Check your posture by connecting to your core muscles and step up with your left foot, making sure your heel is firmly on the step.
- Follow your left with your right foot, then step back down, left then right.
- Continue with this pattern—left up, right up, left down, right down—for the required length of time.
- * Change to lead on your right leg halfway through.

Hints & Tips

- To achieve the correct speed, work at around 25–30 steps per minute. Use a stopwatch so that you can count your steps. Moving faster will increase intensity, which is fine so long as you can maintain correct technique.
- If holding dumbbells, be aware of your shoulder and upper back core muscles—aim always to stand tall.
- To progress, increase your step height to 12 inches and/or increase the dumbbells' weight.

skip jumps

Aim: To simulate a skipping action as if using a jump rope, increasing cardiovascular output to a medium intensity.

Focus: Imagine you are skipping over a rope. Keep your foot action low to the ground, so that you can work on getting your skipping speed up and maintain better core control.

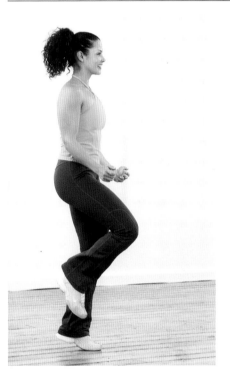 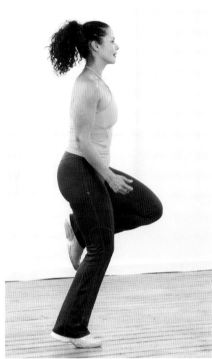

Method

- Place an imaginary rope in your hands and turn your wrists and forearms in a forward circular motion.
- Lift your right knee. Hop on your left foot as you bring your right heel down in front. This is your hop-skip action, that is, lift right knee, hop on left, and strike down with right heel in front.
- Rotate your forearms forward once for each hop–skip action.
- As your right heel strikes down, place your weight onto your right foot and repeat the pattern by lifting your left knee, hopping onto your right foot, and striking down with your left heel.
- Keep repeating, right then left, for the time indicated on your chosen workout.

Hints & Tips

- If you have a jump rope you can use one. However, be careful if skipping inside your home! And if you haven't done it for a while, it's not so easy as you may remember.
- Aim to keep your back tall and your core muscles connected throughout the exercises.
- To progress, speed up the skipping action by taking out the hop and jumping straight from one heel in front to the next.

front kick

Aim: To use a martial-arts kicking action to increase your energy output, while also developing tone and strength in your leg and buttock muscles.

Focus: Focus on kicking to a fixed point no higher than your own thigh height. When kicking, aim to push through using the muscle in the front of your thigh (Quadriceps).

Method

- Begin in what is known as "fighting stance"—left foot in front, right foot behind, fists up to cover your face and upper torso—your left fist should be high enough to cover your face and your right fist to cover your chest.
- Lift your right knee up high, hold and balance, and connect to your core. Your left knee should be slightly bent and toes turned slightly out.

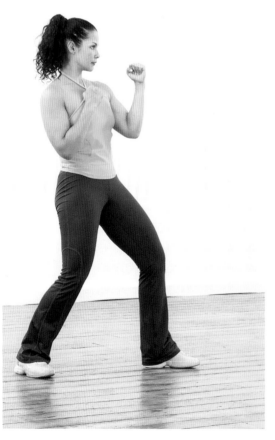

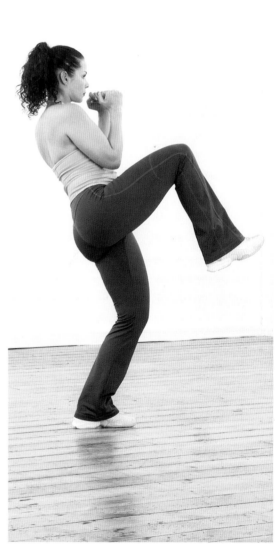

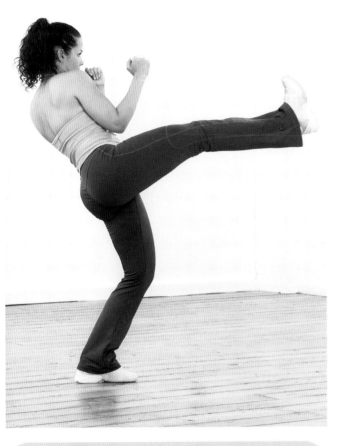

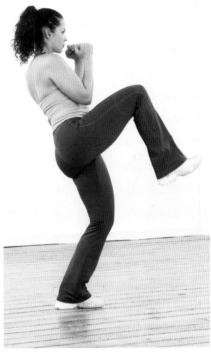

Hints & Tips

- Imagine you have an opponent. Aim your kick to the thigh just above their knee.
- Never throw your lower leg out as you kick. Use muscle control, keeping the knee slightly bent at all times.
- Pulling back into the knee lift position after you have kicked will help to protect the knee and use more leg muscles.
- If you have any knee concerns, do the knee lift without the kick.
- To progress, increase the speed of your kicks, taking 3–6 seconds per kick. You can start to aim higher, as shown in the picture. However, build up slowly and carefully.

- Return your foot back to the starting position and practice knee lifts only.
- Once you are ready to try the kick, extend at the right knee, pushing the ball of your foot forward as if trying to kick open a door.
- Pull back into a knee lift position, hold, and balance.
- Take your foot back to the starting position ready to kick again
- Repeat 8–10 kicks with your left leg, taking 8–12 seconds to complete a kick. Change sides.

rocking horse

Aim: To use the step to increase energy output while exercising the glutes.

Focus: As you lift onto the step, squeeze your butt and connect to your core abdominals as your leg extends back.

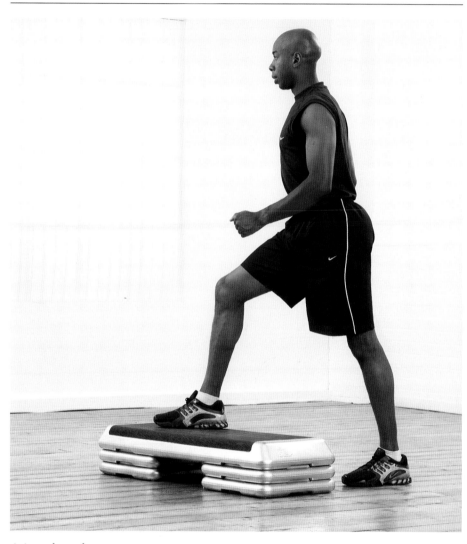

Method

- Use a step about 8–12 inches high and stand in front with your feet within a foot's length from the step.
- Step up with your right foot onto the step.
- Lift your torso high, connect to your core and extend from your left hip joint to bring your left leg behind, squeezing your buttocks.

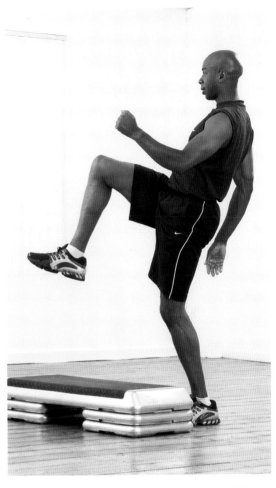

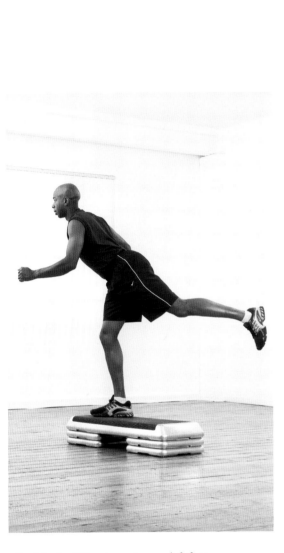

- Rock back off the step onto your left foot.
- Lift your right knee, keeping the left knee soft and your back tall.
- Repeat the action, rocking forward but lifting tall, onto the step again.
- Repeat and change legs halfway through as indicated on your chosen workout.

Hints & Tips

- Be careful that you lower back does not arch as you lift and squeeze your buttocks. Keep working on your core abdominals.
- Aim to work at around 25–30 movements per minute, use a stopwatch to time yourself so that you can count your moves. Going faster will increase the intensity, which is fine so long as you can maintain the correct technique.
- To progress, as you come up onto the step and extend one leg behind, add a jump, lifting up tall.
- Ensure that the whole of your foot comes into contact with the step, especially when you add the jump to progress.

step knee lifts

Aim: To use the step to increase energy output and engage core muscles.
Focus: Concentrate on big, strong moves, while using your core to increase muscle energy output.

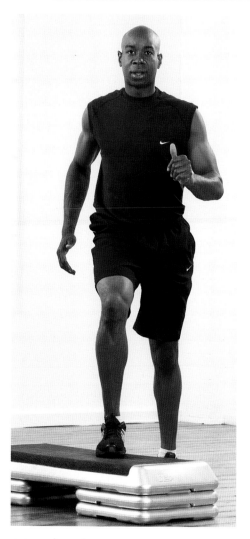 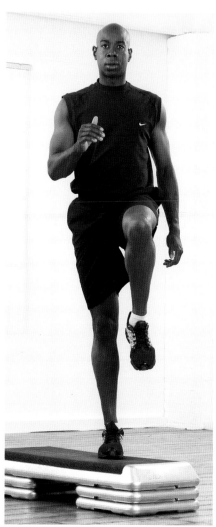

Method

- Use a step around 8–12 inches high and stand in front with your feet within a foot's length from the step.
- Step up onto the step with your right foot, making sure that the whole of your foot lands on the step.
- Lift your left knee and pull up tall, reconnecting to your core muscles.
- Now step back with your left foot, down on to the floor.

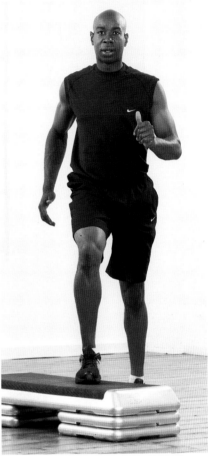

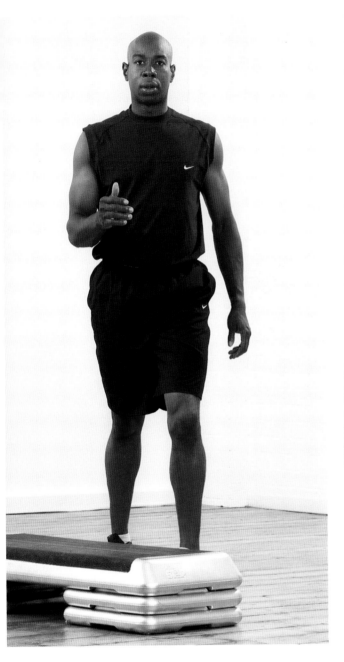

Hints & Tips

- Make sure the whole of your foot comes into contact with the step.
- To get the right speed, aim to work at around 25–30 movements per minute, use a stopwatch to time yourself so that you can count your moves. Going faster will increase the intensity, which is fine so long as you can maintain the correct technique.
- To progress, increase the length of your lunge back, lowering your torso closer to the floor. Keep your spine in its natural postural position and connect to your core.

- Keeping your chest lifted, transfer your weight into your left foot, step behind with your right foot into an easy lunge position.
- Your movement pattern is step up right, lift left knee, step down left onto the floor, lunge behind right.
- Repeat the action, changing sides to bring your left foot onto the step.

step in and punch

Aim: To use punching and stepping actions in a controlled but fast and strong rhythm, producing an increased energy output.

Focus: Imagine you have an opponent and you are going to quickly step toward them, punch once to the chin and once to the chest, and then pull back quickly out of harm's way.

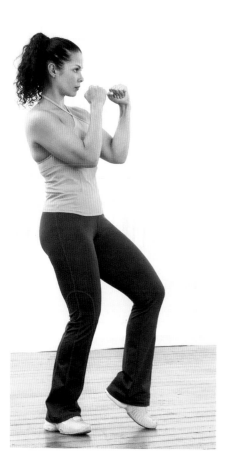
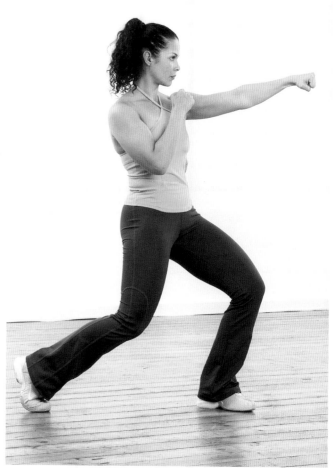

Method

- Start in "fighting stance"—left foot in front, right foot behind, fists up to cover your face and upper torso—your left fist should be high enough to cover your face and your right fist to cover your chest.
- Take a step forward, right foot followed by left, and extend your left arm out to aim a punch at your imaginary opponent's chin.
- Pull back with your left arm and, as you do, draw your right hip and arm through to aim a punch at your imaginary opponent's chest.

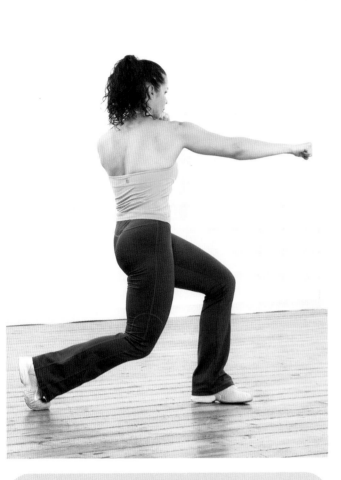

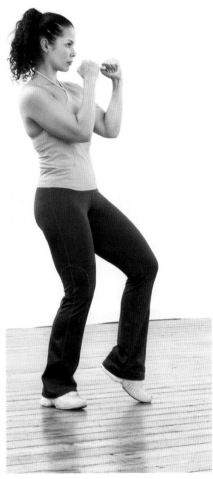

Hints & Tips

- When punching, avoid closing out your elbow joints. Keep the arm slightly bent at all times and aim to use muscle control—imagine your arm is moving through water.
- The bigger the step you take, the harder the move will be. Use big movements, but always aim to keep your back tall, core connected.
- Never lean your torso forward. Keep your spine vertical and create more length by taking bigger steps and bringing your right hip forward on the second punch.
- To progress, increase your speed to 2 seconds per movement and add a leap as you move in with your first punch.

- Use your right hip to bring your right side uppermost and bend at both knees to lower your arm into the chest height, punch position.
- Pull back with your right side and take a step back, left foot followed by right, back into your "fighting stance."
- Repeat the movement 10–15 times and change sides.
- Aim to take 4 seconds to complete the move in the following rhythm: step in and punch left arm—then right—step back right—step back left.

step lunges

Aim: To use the step to increase energy output and effort in your lunges.

Focus: Work with strong movements. Keep your posture in check and connect to your core to keep your lower back safe as you lunge.

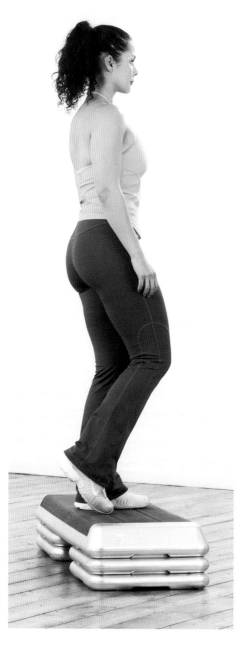

Method

- Use a step around 8–12 inches high. Stand with the whole of both of your feet firmly on top of your step.
- Take a step back with your right foot, lowering back to touch the floor with the ball of your foot only.
- If you find it hard to balance, extend both arms out in front as you lunge.
- Work on your abdominal, shoulder, and back core muscles to maintain correct posture.

Hints & Tips

- Lunges off a step place extra demands on the lower leg muscles and tendons. Keep the heel off the floor as you lunge and pay particular attention to the calf stretches in your cool-down.
- To get the right speed, aim to work at around 30 lunges per minute; use a stopwatch.
- To progress, increase the length of your lunge away from your step. For an additional challenge, add a jump as you change from lunging right to left.

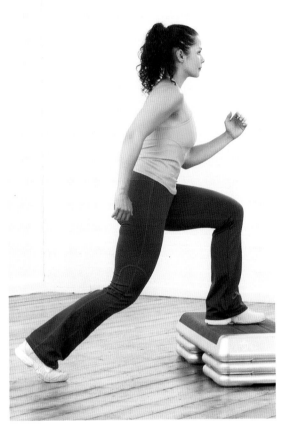

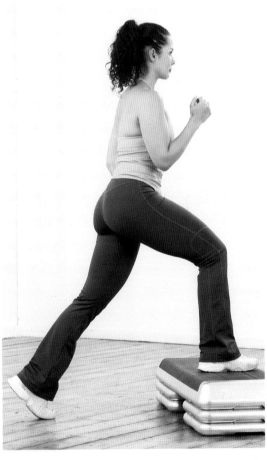

- Lift your right foot back on top of the step, bringing your arms back by your side.
- Repeat the action with your left.
- Keep repeating, alternating from right to left, that is, lunge back right, lunge back left, for the time allotted in your chosen workout.

side to side leaps

Aim: To use a wide but low jumping action for a high cardiovascular (heart and lung) training effect. This is suitable for short bursts of high intensity.

Focus: Concentrate on strong moves with correct posture. Go for length rather than height as you travel from side to side.

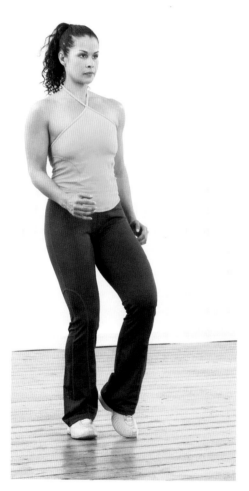
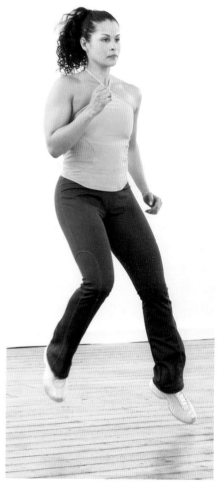

Method

- Start with your feet close, ready to take a step out to the left side.
- Think about your posture and connect to your core.
- To begin, step to the side—left followed by right—without jumping, that is, step to the left with your left foot, then right foot.
- Repeat back to the right, that is, step to the right, right foot then left.
- Repeat this sequence aiming gradually to make your step wider each time.

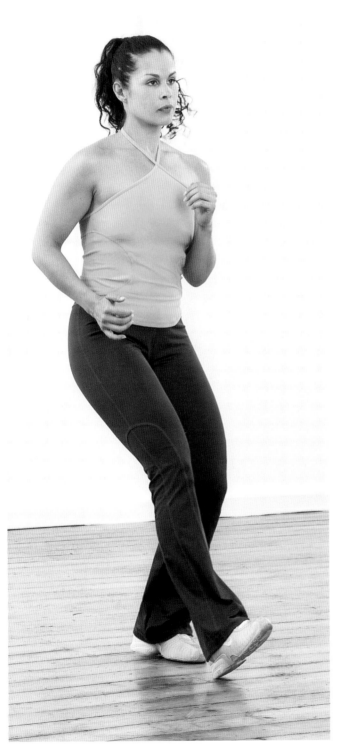

- As you get more confident with the move, start to leap across, side-to-side, rather than just step.
- To complete the movement shown in the picture, leap across left then right, placing your right heel down in front.
- Repeat back to the left.

Hints & Tips

- This is a high-intensity exercise and therefore must be built up carefully. If you find it too much, stick to the step across only, as described.
- Aim to work at a speed of roughly 1 leap or 1 step per second. As you improve, aim to increase to 90 leaps per minute.
- To progress, increase the length of your leap and, ensuring you maintain good posture, increase your speed.

side and back lunges

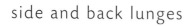

Aim: To generate a moderate cardiovascular training effect, bringing your energy levels into your fat-burning zone.

Focus: Use strong, definite moves, staying low to the ground. Concentrate on good posture and core control throughout.

Method

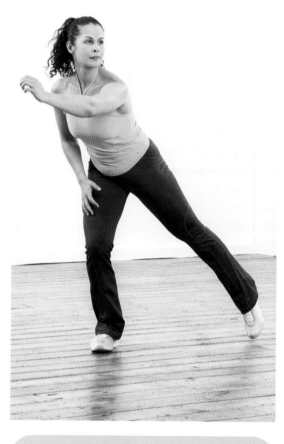

- Step out with your right leg to the side, then your left, then alternate.
- As you step out with your right foot, shift your body slighty to face left, and vice versa.
- Use your arms as shown in the picture—step side right, bring your right arm out in front. Do the same on the left side.
- Repeat this 20 times on each leg.

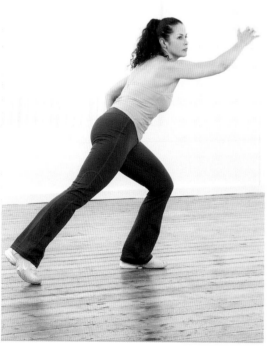

Hints & Tips

- It is important to keep your heel off the ground as you lunge. Touch down and push off from the ball of your foot only.
- Always keep your chest lifted throughout the lunging movement, not forgetting to connect to your shoulder, back and abdominal core areas.
- To progress, jump rather than step to the side and back.

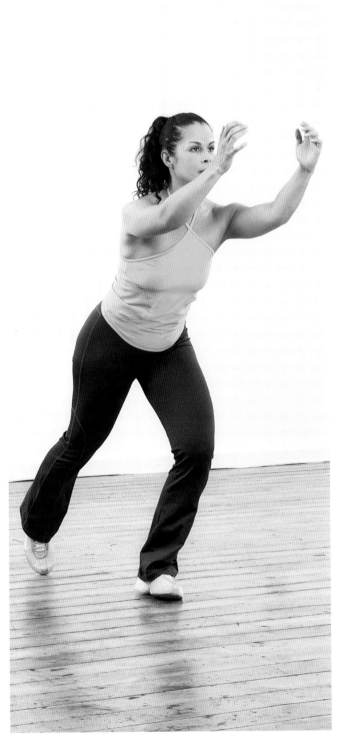

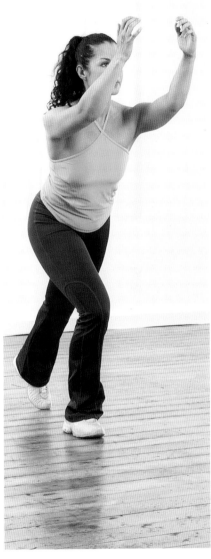

- Next, keeping your body facing front, take big steps behind you, alternating your right and left leg.
- Repeat 20 times on each leg.
- Continue to repeat 20 of each movement for the time specified on your chosen workout.

squat and jump

Aim: To burn fat through a moderate to high cardiovascular (heart and lung) activity, that also adds strength, tone, and power to the legs (Hamstrings and Quadriceps) and glutes.
Focus: Concentrate on sitting back into the squatting action, lifting through using your butt rather than just your thighs.

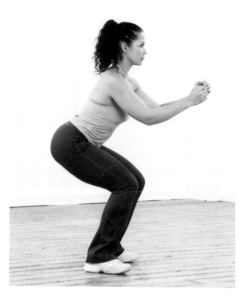

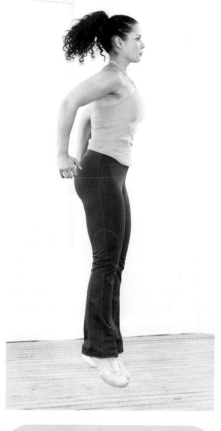

Method

- Stand with your feet wider than hip-width apart.
- Connect to your core and, squatting back, put your weight into your heels.
- Use your arms to counterbalance by extending them forward as you squat.
- Lift back up in a strong, powerful move, squeezing your buttocks as you lift.
- Lower again and repeat this action once, then lower again into a squat for a third time.
- On this third squat, lift, jump, and pull your arms back as both feet lift off the floor.
- Land carefully, using your legs as shock absorbers, bending at the knee to lower into a fourth squat.
- Your movement pattern is: squat-lift, squat-lift, squat-jump, squat-lift.
- Move through the squats quickly. To help maintain good technique, do not squat deeper than you can control and keep good posture and core muscle connection.
- Keep repeating this pattern for the time given in your chosen workout.

Hints & Tips

- You need to perform this movement at a constant pace and rhythm. Aim to complete one cycle in around 4 seconds, or 15 movements per minute.
- To progress, add more jumps to the movement pattern, for example, squat-lift, squat-jump, squat-jump, squat-lift.

Cardio Circuit—Advanced

run ups

Aim: Gradually to increase cardiovascular (heart and lung) output for continuous fat burning exercises.

Focus: Careful foot placement, speed, and posture are important. Focus on making sure each foot lands firmly on the step.

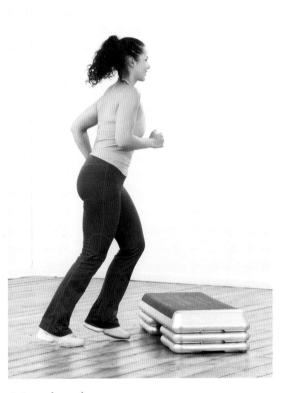 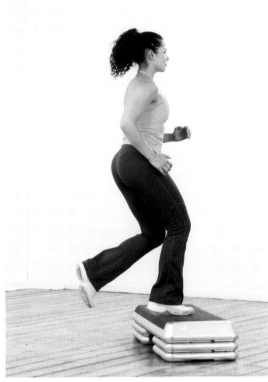

Method

- Use a step 8–10 inches in height. Stand within your foot's distance from the step.
- Check your posture by connecting to your core muscles and run onto the step with your right foot, making sure your heel is firmly on the step.
- Follow your right with your left foot, then run off, right then left.
- Continue with this pattern—right up, left up, right down, left down—for the required length of time.
- Change to lead with your other leg halfway through the allotted time.

Hints & Tips

- If you find that this movement places stress on your lower leg (calf muscles), then start by running up and stepping down.
- Start working at around 30 Run Ups per minute—use a stopwatch to keep time. Going faster will increase intensity, which is fine, so long as you can maintain the correct technique.
- To progress, increase the step height up to 12 inches, working at faster but still, as always, controlled speeds.

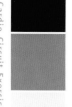

lunges off the side of the step

Aim: To use the step to increase energy output for continuous fat burning training.
Focus: Work with strong movements. Keep your posture in check and connect to your core to keep your lower back safe as you leap and lunge.

Method

- Use a step around 8–12 inches high. Stand in the middle of your step, facing lengthwise, both of your feet firmly on the step.
- Take a step out to the side with your right foot, lowering to the side to touch the floor with just the ball of your foot.

Hints & Tips

- Keep the heel off the ground as you lunge to the floor.
- Lunges off a step can place extra demands on the lower leg muscles and tendons. To counteract this, pay close attention to the calf stretches in your cool-down exercises.
- To get the right speed, aim to work at around 30–40 lunges per minute. Use a stopwatch to time yourself as you count your steps.
- To increase the intensity, jump higher over the step, ensuring that your whole foot lands safely on top of the step each time.

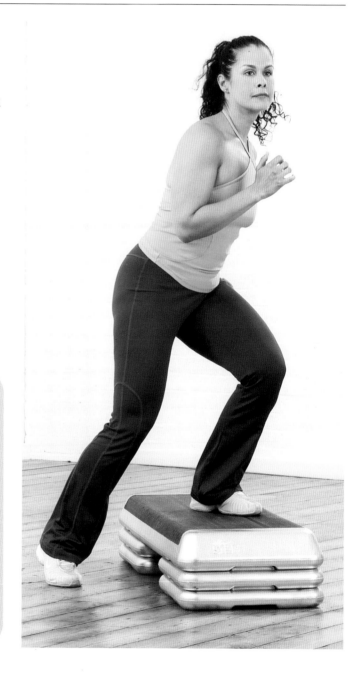

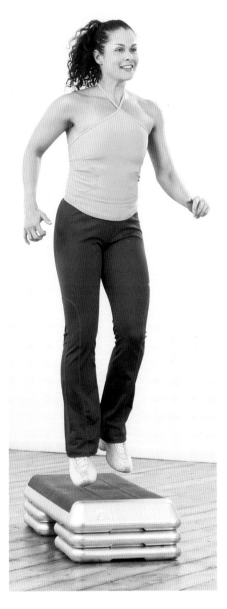

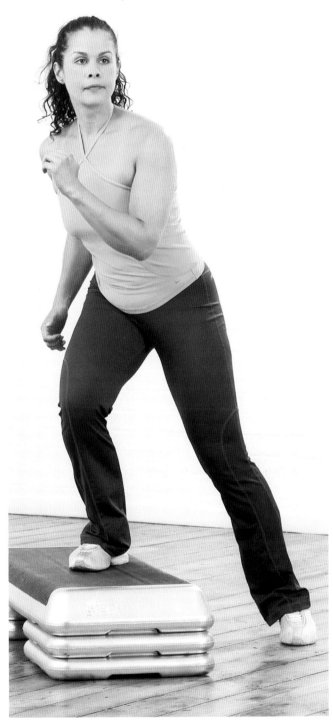

- Work on your abdominal, shoulder, and back core muscles to keep correct posture.
- Lift up by leaping high to bring your right foot back on top of the step.
- Repeat the action with your left.
- Keep repeating, alternating from right to left, that is, lunge back right, lunge back left, for the time allotted in your chosen workout.

round house kick

Aim: To use a kicking action employed in several martial arts to increase your energy output, while also developing tone and strength in your leg and butt muscles.

Focus: Focus on kicking to a fixed point no higher than your own thigh height. When kicking, aim to push through using the front thigh muscle (Quadriceps) and back of your thigh.

Method

- Start in the "fighting stance"—left foot in front, right foot behind, fists up to cover your face and upper torso.
- Swivel on the ball of your right foot and bring your right knee up high to the front, toes pointing down.
- Your right hip should now be facing the front. Your left knee should be slightly bent and toes turned out to the side.
- Hold and balance, connect to your core. Return your foot back to the starting position and practice some knee lifts only.

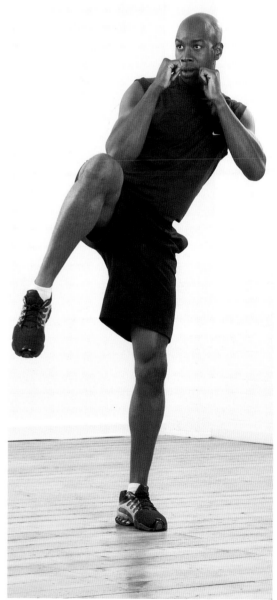
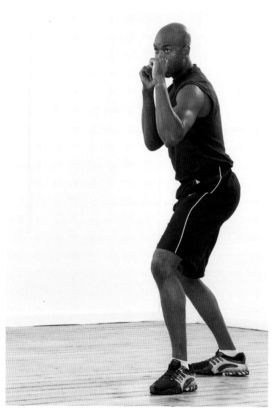

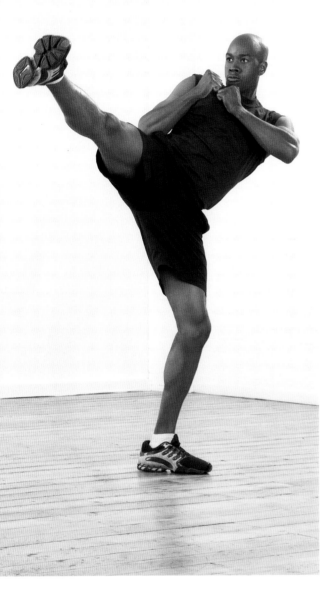

Hints & Tips

- Imagine you have an opponent. Aim your kick to the side of their thigh, just above their knee.
- Be careful not to over-extend at the knee joint. Keep the knee slightly bent at all times.
- Pulling back into the lifted knee position after you have kicked will help to protect the knee and use more muscles in your legs.
- If you have any knee concerns, just do the knee lift without the kick.
- To progress, increase the speed of your kicks, taking 4–6 seconds per kick. You can also start to aim a little higher, as shown in the picture. However, build up slowly and carefully to this.

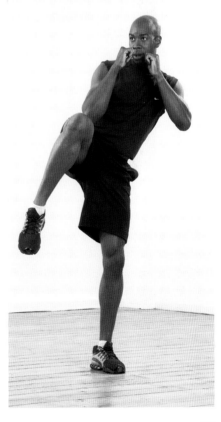

- Once you are ready to try the kick, lean to the left side, keeping your back straight.
- Extend at the right knee joint, aiming to kick an imaginary opponent on the thigh with the front of your foot. Allow your left foot to swivel on the ball of the foot toward the back.
- Pull back without snapping out at the knee, hold, and balance.
- Take your foot back to the starting position, ready to kick again.
- Repeat 8–10 kicks with your left leg, taking 8–12 seconds between kicks. Change sides.

jump up and run around

Aim: To produce a moderate cardiovascular (heart and lung) training effect and improve leg strength.

Focus: Aim to move quickly and continuously around the step. When jumping, concentrate on using muscles in your legs and butt to land safely on and off the step.

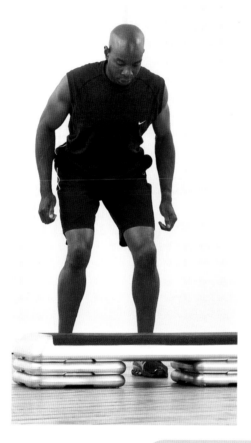
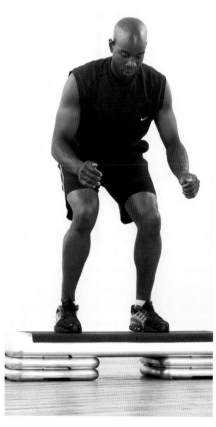

Method

- Stand within a foot's distance from the step. Take your arms behind you and bend the knees to prepare to jump.
- Connect to your core and jump up onto the step with both feet firmly on top, knees bent.

Hints & Tips

- When jumping, give yourself a soft landing by bending the knees and sitting your weight back. This will minimize stress to the knee joint and increase the strength of your legs and buttock muscles.
- To keep you balanced on top of the step as you land, use your shoulder, back, and abdominal core muscles to keep your back tall and weight evenly distributed.
- To progress, increase the height of your step and aim to run a little faster.

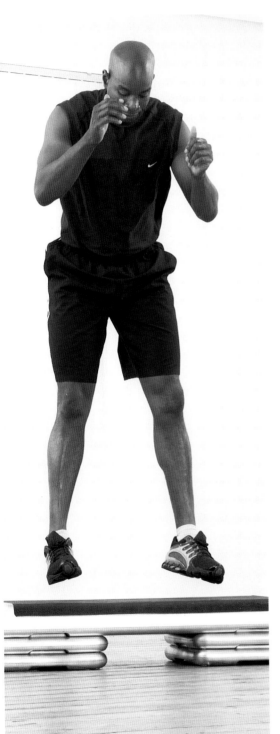

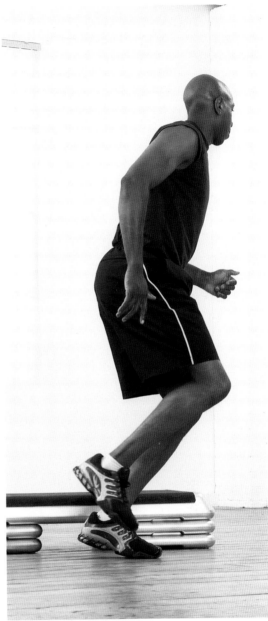

- Jump off the step to the front and run around to the back, turning to your left.
- Repeat the movement, jumping on to and off the step, except this time, turn right as you run around. Repeat, alternating the direction of your run.

ski jumps

Aim: To add a high intensity movement for working up to peak intensity in cardio circuit activities, and as a high intensity mode in interval-training workouts.

Focus: Aim to lift up high as you jump, concentrating on using muscles in your legs (Hamstrings and Quadriceps) and bottom to land safely.

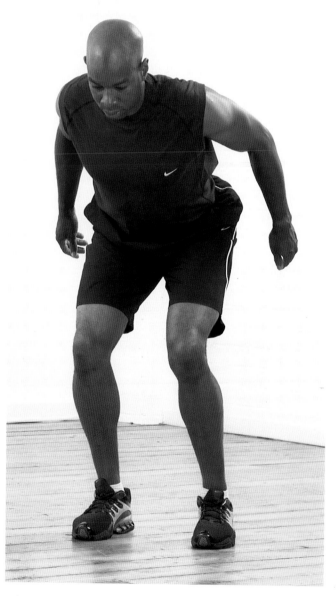

Method

- Place your feet hip-width apart in parallel lines.
- Sit back into a shallow squat position, arms behind as if planting ski poles behind you.
- Jump up, shifting your body to the right. Connect to your core and lift your arms as you jump to help propel you up and over to the left.

Hints & Tips

- The higher you jump and lower you land, the more potential stress you will place on your back and knee joints. To avoid this, always connect to your core and sit with your weight back, keeping your knees behind your toes as you land.
- To progress, jump higher and land into a full squat position.

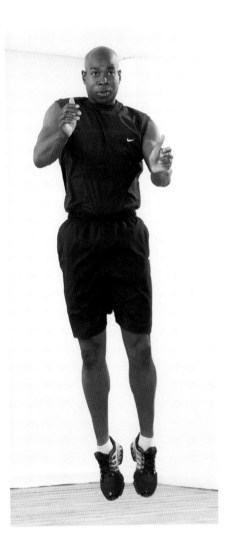

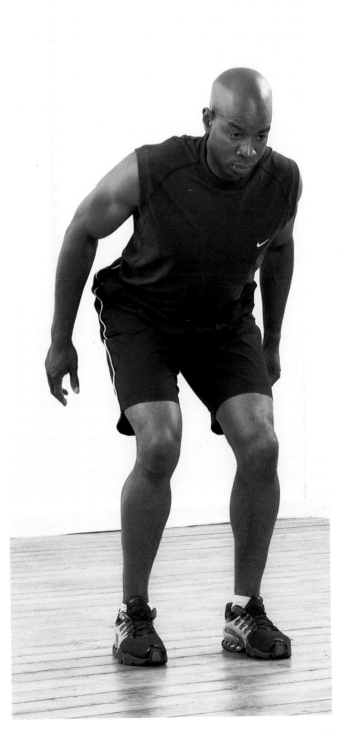

- Land with your feet parallel, in a diagonal line to the front.
- Bend your knees, sitting back into a squat position as you land, arms back behind you.
- Immediately lift up and jump again, this time landing to the right, on a diagonal line to the front.

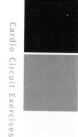

side jump lunges

Aim: To generate a moderate to high cardiovascular training effect, bringing your energy levels into your fat burning intensity zone.

Focus: Use strong, definite moves. Concentrate on good posture and core control.

Method

- Start by stepping out to the side and slightly behind you, using your right foot.
- Place your weight on to the ball of your foot only.
- Focus on your core muscles, keeping your shoulders back and down, chest lifted and abdominals pulled in.
- Push off from the right foot and jump towards the left.

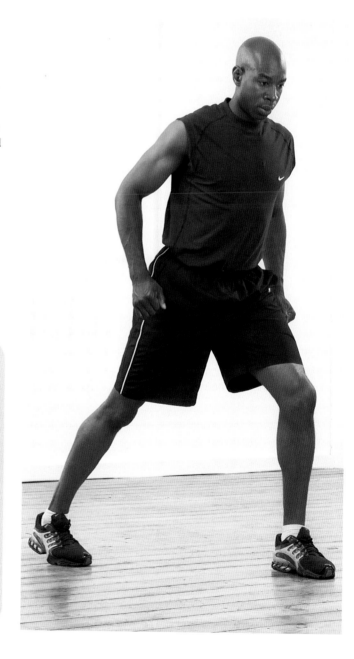

Hints & Tips

- Keep your heel off the ground as you lunge. Touch down and push off from the ball of your foot only.
- If you are working on a continuous program such as the Fat Burner Cardio Circuit or the Mix It sessions, don't push yourself too hard. You should be able to move to your next exercise without feeling exhausted. If doing an interval workout you can allow yourself to work a little harder.
- To progress, increase the length of your lunges and height of your jumps. Protect your knee joints by keeping your weight into the heel of your non-lunging foot.

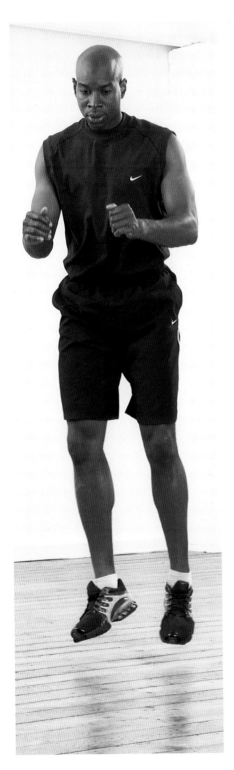

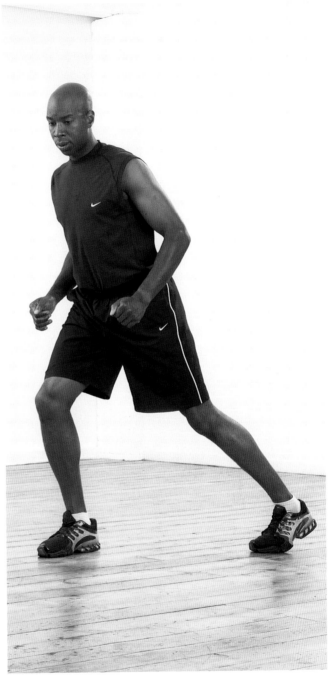

- Land on your right foot and lunge out with your left.
- Repeat changing from left to right. Move at a paceat which you can maintain your posture and correct intensity.

knee leaps on the step

Aim: To use the step to increase energy output through long, large movements.
Focus: Concentrate on big, strong moves, while using your core to increase muscle energy output.

Method

- Use a step about 10–12 inches high. Stand in front with your feet within a foot's length from the step.
- Step up with your left foot, making sure the whole of your foot lands on the step.
- Lift your right knee and leap up, pulling up tall through your back and re-connecting to your core muscles.

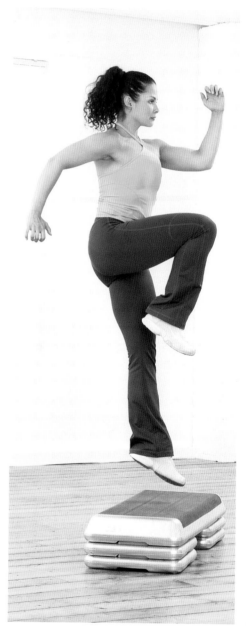

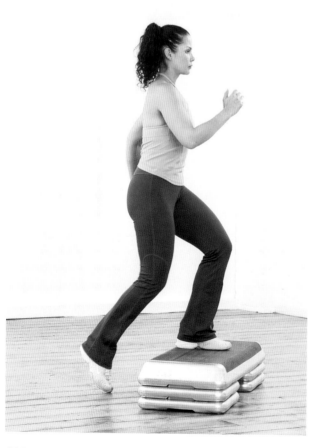

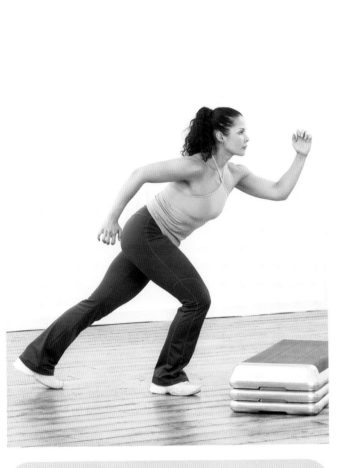

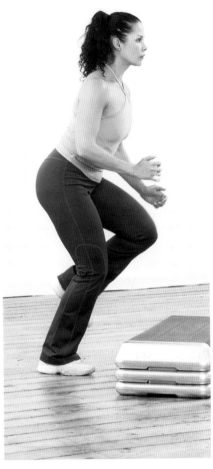

- Step back with your right foot, down onto the floor.
- Keeping your chest lifted, weight into your right foot, step behind with your left foot into a lunge position.
- Your movement pattern is: step up left, leap and lift right knee, step back, right foot onto the floor, lunge behind left.
- Repeat the action, changing sides to bring your right foot onto the step.

Hints & Tips

- Make sure the whole of your foot comes into contact with the step.
- To get the right speed, aim to work at around 30 movements per minute—use a stopwatch to time yourself so that you can count your moves. Going faster will increase the intensity, which is fine, so long as you can maintain the correct technique as described for the time given in the workout.
- To progress, leap higher and increase the length of your lunge back. To do this, bend the knee of your non-lunging leg more to bring your torso closer to the floor. Keep your weight into the heel of the non-lunging leg and maintain your spine's correct position by connecting to your core.

step in, punch, and kick

Aim: To use martial arts-style punching and kicking actions in a controlled, but fast and strong rhythm producing increased energy output.

Focus: Imagine you have an opponent you are going to quickly step in toward, punch once to the chin and kick once on the side of the thigh, then you pull back quickly out of harm's way.

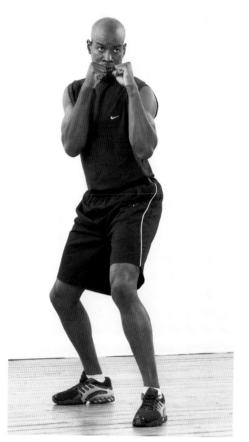 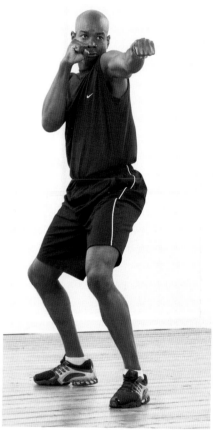

Method

- Start in "fighting stance"—left foot in front, right foot behind, fists up to cover your face and upper torso.
- Take a step forward, left foot followed by right, and extend your left arm out to aim a punch at your imaginary opponent's chin.
- Draw your left arm back and, putting your weight into your right foot, swivel on the ball of your foot to turn your right foot out and lift your left knee, toes pointing down.
- Make sure your right knee is soft and toes are turned out to the side.
- Take two steps backward.
- Repeat this action, that is, step in, punch, lift knee, and take two steps back, until you feel comfortable with your technique.

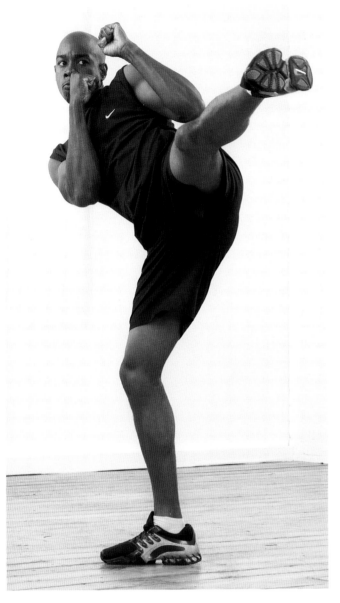

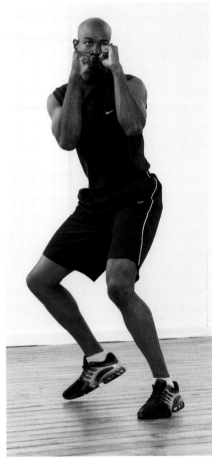

- When and if you feel ready, add the kick. Extend at the left knee joint, aiming to kick an imaginary opponent on the thigh with the front of your foot. Allow your right foot to swivel on the ball of the foot toward the back. Bring your leg back into the knee-lift position, being careful not to jerk or snap the knee joint. Lower your leg and take 2 steps back in a shuffling action.
- Repeat the movement 10–15 times and change sides. Aim to take 4 seconds to complete the move in the following rhythm: step in and punch left arm, round house kick, take two shuffles back.

Hints & Tips

- Be very careful when punching and kicking not to lock out your joints. Keep the knee and elbow slightly bent at all times and aim to use muscle control. Imagine your arms and legs are moving through water.
- The bigger the steps you take, the harder the move will be. Use big movements, but always aim to keep your back tall, shoulders back and down, and abs pulled in.
- To progress, increase your speed to 2 seconds per movement and add a leap as you move in with your punch.

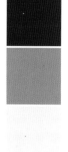

leap over the step

Aim: To use long movements to bring about a high intensity cardiovascular effect. This will bring you into the upper regions of your fat burning zone.

Focus: Concentrate on careful placement of your feet on top of the step and using big movements to ensure you reach the other end.

Method

- Place your self at the right end of the step and within a foot's distance from it.
- Stand tall and connect to your core.
- Step up with your left foot toward the middle of the step.
- Leap up, pushing weight into your left foot and jump to transfer your weight onto your right leg.
- As you jump up you should be aiming to travel sideways across the step; so that your right foot lands on top of the step but toward the left end.
- Step down with your left foot onto the left end of the step, followed by your right.
- Repeat, going back to the right side.

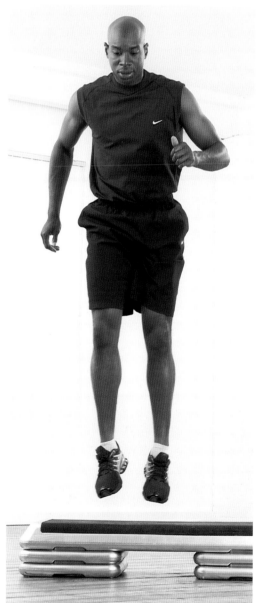

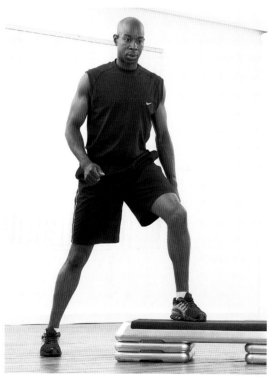

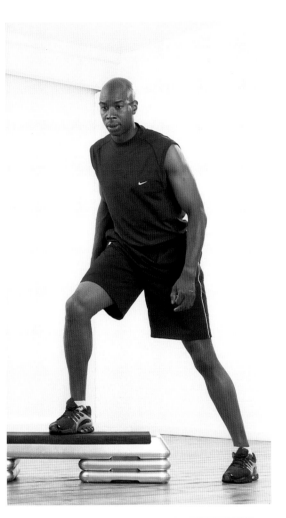

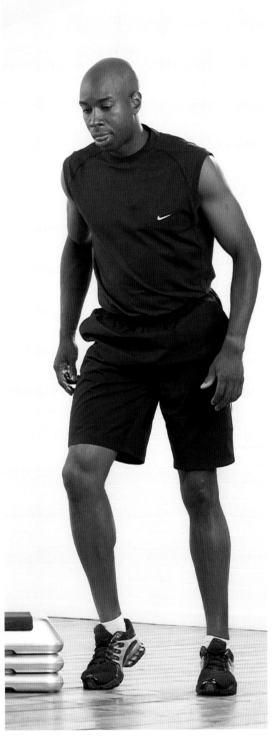

Hints & Tips

- As you are traveling across a narrow area you need to pay particular attention to your balance. Avoid leaning forward by always thinking about your posture and connecting to your core.
- With sideways movements it's important to lift up your feet and put them down carefully to avoid injuring your ankle. Do this movement in front of a mirror so that you can check where your feet are going without having to lean forward to look down.
- To progress, move a little faster, take bigger leaps, and lift up with your arms as you leap.

high step ups

Aim: To increase the heart rate using large stepping movements, while adding strength to the main muscles in the legs and butt.

Focus: Concentrate on correct posture and lifting up through your butt as you push through your heel and stand tall on the step.

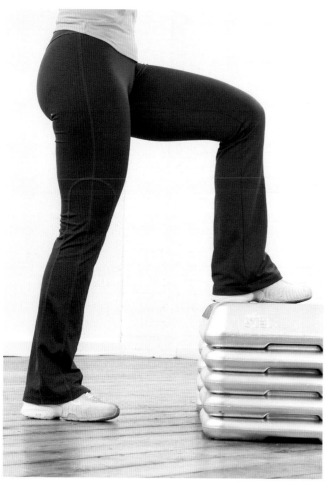

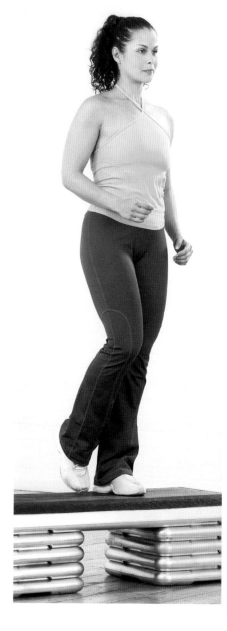

Method

- Use a 12–16 inch high step. Your leg length should dictate the height of the step: when you step up, your leg should not go lower than a 90-degree bend.

106

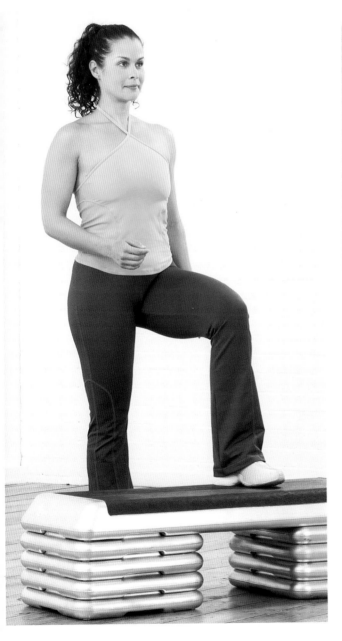

Hints & Tips

- These steps ups should be performed at a pace at which you feel you can maintain good posture and core control. Aim to work slowly but fast enough that you feel yourself going into the right intensity to burn fat.
- If holding dumbbells, make sure you work extra hard on your shoulder and upper back core muscles to keep the shoulders back and down. Aim always to stand tall.
- To progress, increase the step height, ensuring you can still step up with a comfortable bend at the knee joint (no lower than 90 degrees). Alternatively, hold heavier dumbbells.

- Stand just within your foot's distance from the step.
- Check your posture by connecting to your core muscles and step up with your left foot, making sure your heel is firmly on the step.
- Follow your left with your right foot, pushing through the heel of your left foot and using your butt to stand tall on the step. Step back down, right then left.
- Change to lead on your left leg halfway through the allotted time.

Cool-Down Stretches

The following stretches have been designed for you to use at the end of your workouts. There are also selected exercises that you will use in your Core Strength and Length Session.

Unlike any of the exercises given in this book, the cool-down stretches will not have a direct bearing on your ability to burn fat. Stretches, however, are a highly important part of any fitness routine and it is a mistake to leave them out because while these exercises may not have a direct bearing on your ability to burn fat, they do have a direct bearing on your ability to work out.

By including well thought-out stretching exercises in your fat burner program you will increase the safety and efficiency of all of your other exercises, enabling you to stick to your program and ultimately burn more fat.

As well as helping you to keep up your workouts each week, stretching will also give you the following benefits: increased flexibility, increased joint mobility, injury prevention, improved posture, improved shape, better body balance, stress relief, and a calming end to your workout.

Aim to do each stretch, in sequence, at the end of your workout. If you are stretching outside, for example, in the park or the back yard, you can omit the stretches that require you to use a ball. However, make sure that you do include these stretches the following day, either through doing your Core Strength and Length routine or an indoor workout where you use the stretches in your cool-down.

Short Stretch Routine

Do this when you are short on time, making sure you do a full stretch the next day:

1. Calf Stretch 1
2. Wall Chest Stretch
3. Deep Hip (Glute) Stretch
4. Hamstring Stretch
5. Back Rotation Stretch
6. Knee Hug
7. Hip Flexor And Front Thigh Stretch

For each stretch follow these vital points:
- Hold each stretch for a minimum of 30 seconds.
- Listen to your body and ensure that you feel the stretch as indicated by the "Focus" given for each exercise.
- Always ease into a stretch by breathing out and moving gently.
- Never bounce, or use forceful or jerky movements.
- Only move onto the progressions if you don't feel much of a stretch and know that your muscles are quite flexible.
- Connect to your core; holding good posture will ensure you are working the right area.
- If you feel you have an area that is particularly tight, go back and stretch this area a second time.

Cool-Down Stretch

lower leg (calf) stretch 1

Aim: To stretch out the main calf muscle, called the Gastrocnemius.

Focus: This muscle runs from above the knee, down into the big tendon (the Achilles) that inserts into your heel bone. Concentrate on the feeling from the back of your knee down toward your Achilles tendon.

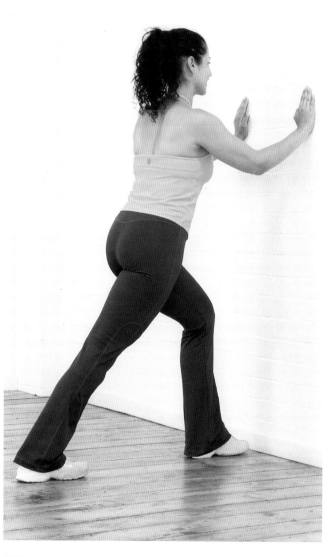

Method

- Place your hands up against a wall, right leg extended behind, left leg bent in front.
- Make sure your body is in a straight line, core muscles connected.
- Take a breath in and, as you breathe out, bend your elbows and your front knee, pushing your body weight forward until you feel a stretch.
- Hold for 30 seconds, continuing to take slow, deep breaths. Change sides.

Hints & Tips

- It is important to lean in with the whole body. Push forward from your hips keeping your back tall, core muscles connected.
- For a deeper stretch, place the ball of your right foot on a rolled towel.

lower leg (calf) stretch 2

Aim: To stretch the deeper calf muscle, called the Soleus. This attaches to the top of your lower leg bone (tibia) and into the lower leg tendon (Achilles).
Focus: Concentrate on a stretch feeling low down in your leg towards your Achilles tendon and heel bone.

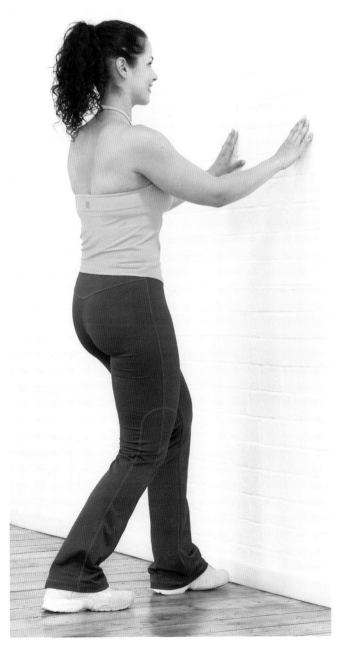

Method

- Stand closer to the wall than in the first stretch.
- Your right foot needs to be behind, left foot in front with about a foot's length between them.
- Take a breath in and, as you breathe out, sink your weight back into the heel of your right foot, bending both knees.
- Hold for 30 seconds, continuing to take slow deep breaths. Change sides.

Hints & Tips

- Aim to keep your back tall and allow your right knee to come forward as you move into the stretch.
- For a deeper stretch, as for the first calf stretch place the ball of your right foot on a rolled towel.

deep hip (glute) stretch

Aim: To stretch out deep muscles in the hip joint. This includes your smaller buttock muscles, the Gluteus Medius, as well as other muscles that allow your hip to rotate.

Focus: Concentrate on a stretch feeling deep in your hip and running slightly down the back of your leg.

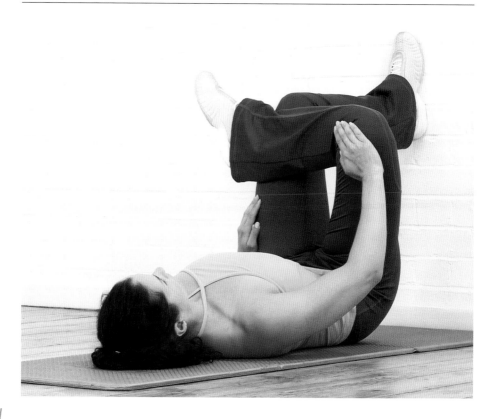

Method

- Lie with your back on the floor close enough to a wall to allow you to place your left foot against the wall with your knee bent at 90 degrees.
- Make sure that you butt is firmly on the floor. Connect to your core abdominal muscles and press your pelvis down. If you can't, then you need to shift farther away from the wall.
- Cross your right foot over the front of your left thigh.
- Take a breath and as you breathe out, gently press the heel of your hand against the inside of your right knee to push you leg farther out to the side.
- Hold for 30 seconds, continuing to take relaxing breaths. Change sides.

Hints & Tips

- When crossing your foot in front of your thigh, aim to line up your anklebone with the middle of your thigh, just above your knee.
- Keep your head and shoulders relaxed back on the floor; if your head is uncomfortable, use a folded towel for support.
- To progress, take another breath, draw in your abs, press your pelvis down even farther, aiming to get your back in a natural position, with a little hollow in your lower back.

hamstring stretch

Aim: To stretch the back of the thigh and ease out the calf muscles.
Focus: Concentrate on a stretch feeling running all the way down the back of your leg.

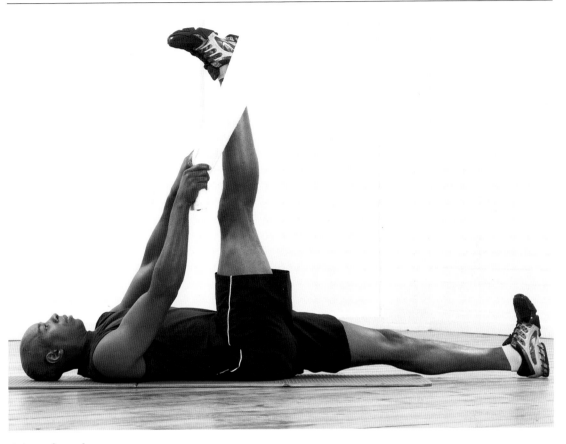

Method

- You will need a towel for this exercise to place around your foot.
- Lie on the floor, both legs outstretched.
- Bring your right leg into your chest and place the towel around the bottom of your foot.
- Take a breath in and as you breathe out, extend your right leg up toward the ceiling.
- Draw in your core abdominals as you do this to protect your lower back.
- Lengthen your left leg away along the floor and aim to keep your bottom on the floor as well.
- Hold for 30 seconds, continuing to take slow, deep breaths. Change sides.

Hints & Tips

- Be careful not to overextend at the knee joint. To protect it, contract the front thigh muscle.
- Keep your head, neck, and shoulders relaxed on the floor as you stretch.
- If your leg starts to shake, bend it back into your chest, relax, and then try to stretch again but with a slight knee bend.
- To progress, take another breath and as you breathe out, gently pull down with the towel to bring your toes closer to your shin.

back rotation stretch

Aim: To stretch out muscles that work diagonally and to the side of the back and waist, including the abductors of the hips.

Focus: Concentrate on a feeling around the middle of your torso between your ribs and pelvis.

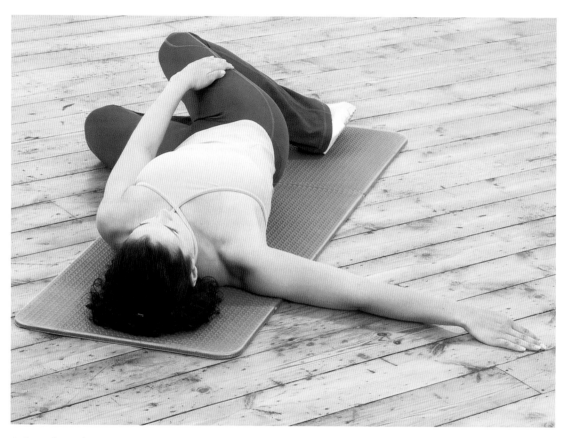

Method

- Lie on your back with both knees bent and your feet flat on the floor.
- Keep your right shoulder firmly on the ground and place your left hand over your right thigh.
- Take a breath and as you breathe out, gently ease your right thigh over to the left, lifting your right hip off the floor. Only go as far as is comfortable for you.
- Hold for 30 seconds, continuing to take slow deep breaths. Change sides.

Hints & Tips

- If you have a stiff back you may find this hard. Listen to your body. Only go as far as you are comfortable. Do smaller stretches but repeat them several times.
- To progress, gently ease your right thigh farther over to the left, making sure your right shoulder stays on the floor.

knee hug

Aim: To stretch out and massage the back muscles that run along the length of your spine.

Focus: Concentrate on relaxing your body into the floor.

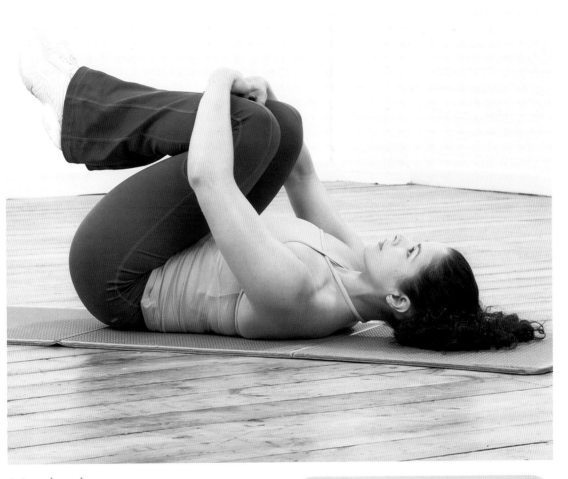

Method

- Lie on your back and take each knee into your chest one at a time.
- Hug both knees into your chest.
- Gently rock from left to right in small movements, gently massaging your back into the floor.
- Hold for 30 seconds, continuing to take slow, deep breaths.

Hints & Tips

- This works better if you are on a deep mat or carpet.
- Each time you breathe out, think about stress flowing away from your body with your breath.
- To progress, place your head on a folded towel. Take a breath in and as you breathe out, roll your head into the towel, bringing your chin into your neck to lengthen the back of the spine all the way up to your head and neck.

lying glute stretch

Aim: To stretch the large buttock muscle (Gluteus Maximus) and the large tendon (Iliotibial band, or ITB) that runs along the outside of your thigh.

Focus: Concentrate on keeping your hips down and square to the floor, so that you feel a stretch coming around the outside of your buttocks, then to the outside of your thigh.

Method

- Lie on your back on the floor.
- Bring your right knee into your chest and hold around the outside of you right knee with your left hand.
- Take a deep breath and as you breathe out gently draw your right knee across to the left until you feel a stretch coming around the outside of your thigh and butt.
- Keep your right hip down on the floor as you do this, connecting to your core abdominal muscles to help keep your pelvis still.
- Hold for 30 seconds, continuing to take slow, deep breaths. Change sides.

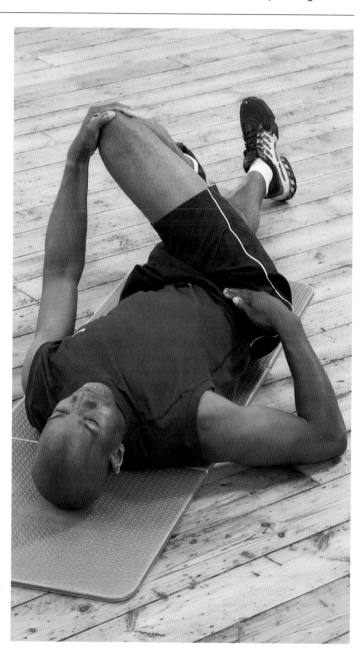

Hints & Tips

- Hold your right hip down by pressing onto it with your right hand.
- If you feel discomfort in your groin as you stretch, ease your knee out to the side to stretch and relieve your groin, hold for 30 seconds, then return to the glute stretch.
- To progress, gently pull over with your knee while actively pulling back with your hip, for a deeper stretch.

116

front thigh and hip flexor stretch

Aim: To stretch out the front of the thigh (Quadriceps) and main hip flexor (Iliacus Psoas).

Focus: Concentrate on using your core abdominal and buttock muscles to bring your hip forward away from your foot, increasing the length of the stretch from your knee and over the hip joint.

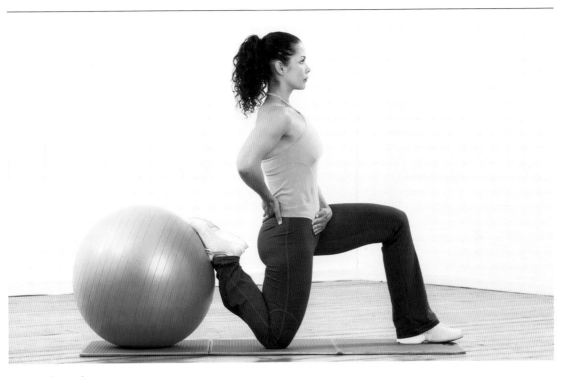

Method

- This stretch works best with a Swiss, or stability ball; but you could use the wall or a bench. Place the ball into the corner of a room so that it cannot roll away.
- Kneel about a foot's distance in front of the ball.
- Using your hands on the floor for balance, place your right foot onto the ball and come up onto the foot of your left leg.
- Bring your torso up into a vertical position and establish your balance, first using the wall for support.
- Once you feel stable in this position, try to take your hands away from the wall and place one hand over your abdomen and the other over the small of your back.
- Take a deep breath in and as you breathe out, gently use your hands to lift your abdomen at the front and push your tailbone down at the back.
- Hold for 30 seconds, continuing to take slow deep breaths. Change sides.

Hints & Tips

- Protect you knee by kneeling on a soft surface; add a towel underneath if it still feels uncomfortable.
- Be very careful of your lower back during this stretch, especially if you are particularly tight at the front of your hip. Aim to protect your lower back by really pulling your abdominals in and using your hands for support. Check in a mirror to make sure that your back does not over-arch.
- For an increased stretch, aim to take your pelvis even farther into a tilted position. (Think of your pelvis as a bucket of water, and you are tipping the water out to the back.)

outer chest stretch

Aim: To stretch out the main chest muscle (Pectoralis major).

Focus: Concentrate on a stretch running from your shoulder joint across to the middle of your chest.

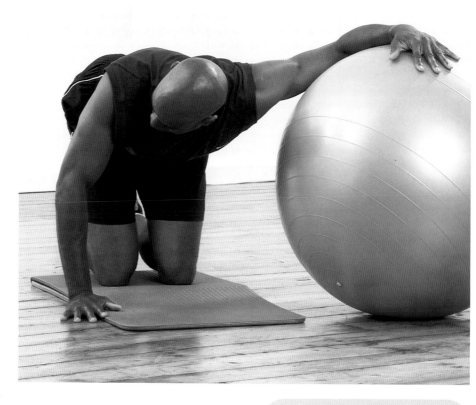

Method

- This stretch works best with a Swiss ball; but you could use a chair or high bench. In a kneeling position, place the ball directly to your left side.
- With the ball positioned to your side, place your arm on top of the ball so that your upper arm is in line with your shoulder and your elbow is bent at 90 degrees.
- Focus on your back and shoulder posture by connecting to your back, shoulder, and deep abdominal core muscles.
- Take a deep breath in and, as you breathe out, open up your shoulder joint at the front by gently pressing your torso down and pulling to the right.
- Hold for 30 seconds, continuing to take slow deep breaths. Change sides.

Hints & Tips

- If you do not feel this stretch in the right place—across your chest— look back at your arm and make sure it is still at right angles and on the top of the ball.
- To help pull in the right direction, turn your head away from the ball as you press down and pull away from the left.
- To progress, contract your back and shoulder core muscles again and aim to pull down and even farther to the left.

deep chest stretch

Aim: To stretch the deep chest muscle (Pectoralis minor).
Focus: Concentrate on a stretch feeling coming from the top of your shoulder and at an acute angle, down to your ribs. This is a deep feeling from seemingly underneath your breastbone.

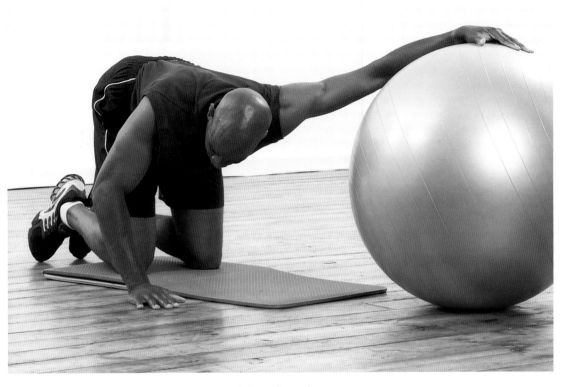

Method

Hints & Tips

- If you do not feel this stretch in the right place, you may need to adjust the angle of the ball. Roll it around slightly, rechecking the stretch each time until you feel a stretch coming diagonally down, from your shoulder to the upper ribs.
- To progress, contract your back and shoulder core muscles and aim to push down and farther, in a direct line, away from the ball.

- This stretch also works best with a Swiss ball; but you could use a chair or high bench. In a kneeling position, place your ball in front of you and slightly out to the right.
- Place your hand and forearm on to of the ball and with your arm straight, check that the ball and your arm is angled at around a 60-degree line from your right side.
- Focus on your back and shoulder posture by connecting to your back, shoulder, and deep abdominal core muscles.
- Take a breath in and, as you breathe out, gentle ease down and pull away from the ball.
- Hold for 30 seconds, continuing to take slow deep breaths. Change sides.

119

neck stretch 1

Aim: To stretch into the neck muscle, the Sternocleidomastoid (which rotates the neck) and an area of the back muscle (Trapezius) that comes around to the side of the neck.

Focus: Concentrate on relaxing your neck, head, and jaw as you feel a stretch coming from behind your ear down to the outer edge of your shoulder.

Method

- Sit tall on your ball and with your right arm lengthened toward the floor.
- Connect to all core muscle areas and place your left hand over your head.
- Take a breath in and, as you breathe out, very gently ease your head over to the right side until you feel a stretch on the left side of your neck.
- Hold for 30 seconds, continuing to take slow, deep breaths. Change sides.

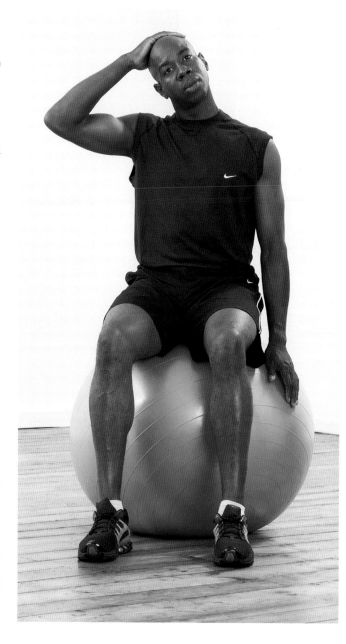

Hints & Tips

- These muscles tend to be very tight. Try to relax as much as you can, as this will help to draw tension away from the neck.
- If your neck remains too tense to stretch, lie back on the floor with your head on a towel and gently roll your head from left to right to help relax your neck muscles.

neck stretch 2

Aim: To stretch into the main part of the back muscle (Trapezius) that comes from the back of your head down to your shoulder blade and spine.

Focus: Concentrate on relaxing your neck, head, and jaw as you feel a stretch coming from the back of your head down toward the back of your shoulder.

Method

- Sit tall on your ball and with your right arm lengthened toward the floor.
- Connect to all core muscle areas and place your left hand over your head.
- Take a breath in and as you breathe out, very gently ease your head over to the right side until you feel a stretch on the left side of your neck and shoulder.
- Hold for 30 seconds, continuing to take slow, deep breaths. Change sides.

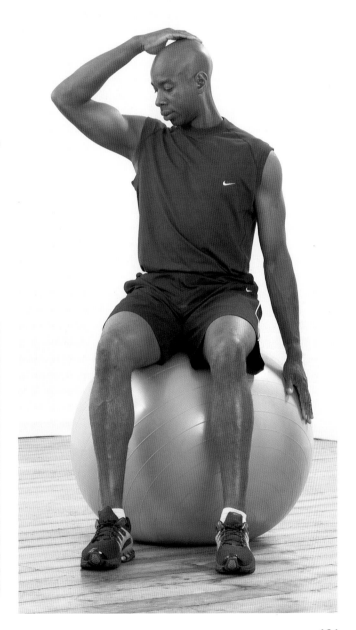

Hints & Tips

- Be extra careful not to over-stretch. Avoid pulling your head forward, aiming to ease it down gently instead.
- If your neck and shoulders feel very tense, do both of your neck stretches every day and not just when you are working out.
- If—and only if—this stretch seems not to be a stretch any more, to progress, place you right hand slightly behind you and rotate out, palms facing front. Contract your back and shoulder muscles to pull your right shoulder farther down. Lengthen your arm and flatten your shoulder blade into the back of your ribs.

rear shoulder and upper back stretch

Aim: To stretch the rear of the shoulder (posterior deltoid), and upper back muscles (Rhomboids. Mid Trapezius and Latissimus Dorsi).

Focus: Concentrate on a stretch running from the back of your shoulder, down to your ribs and waist.

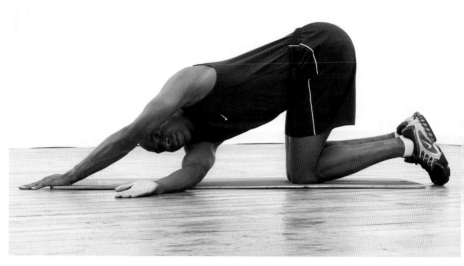

Method

- From an all fours position, place your right arm, palm facing up, underneath you.
- Lower your right shoulder so that your arm reaches through to the left side.
- Angle your right arm slightly up and away from your body.
- Take a deep breath in and, as you breathe out, slowly sink down, lowering your right shoulder farther and sitting back towards your heels.
- Hold for 30 seconds, continuing to take slow deep breaths. Change sides.
- To progress, rotate your whole torso farther to look toward the left side; continue to relax back onto your heels.

Hints & Tips

- If you don't feel this stretch right away, adjust the position of your am and shoulder until you feel a stretch in the area indicated in the focus, above.
- Keep your head relaxed by positioning it between your arms and resting on your right shoulder.

wall chest stretch

Aim: To stretch out the main chest muscle (Pectoralis Major).

Focus: Concentrate on a stretch running from your shoulder joint across to the middle of your chest.

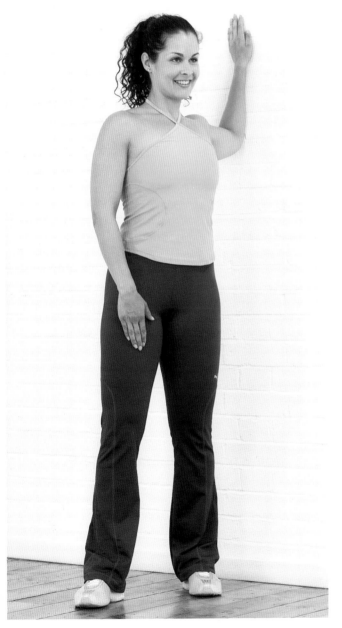

Method

- Stand near to a wall and place your right arm onto the wall.
- Your arm should be bent at 90 degrees with your upper arm in line with your shoulder.
- Focus on your back and shoulder posture by connecting to your back, shoulder, and deep abdominal core muscles.
- Take a deep breath in and, as you breathe out, turn your torso away from your right arm by walking your feet around to the left.
- Hold for 30 seconds, continuing to take slow, deep breaths. Change sides.

Hints & Tips

- If you don't feel this stretch in the right place, that is, across your chest, look back at your arm and make sure it is still at right angles, upper arm at shoulder height
- If you are very tight in this area, be careful not to force too hard against the wall. Take it easy.

The Workouts

In this section you will find 8 different workouts to choose from. Each one begins with an introduction on what the workout is designed to do plus "How to Get Going" step-by-step instructions. Ensure that you read through these steps before beginning the workout. Each workout includes instructions for a warm-up, your 20-minute workout that includes a list of exercises that have appeared in previous sections, and how long each exercise should take to complete.

The main workout is followed by a core strength exercise and your cool-down stretches. One exception to this will be your Core Strength and Length workout where stretches and core exercises are incorporated into the 20-minute workout.

Here is also a quick reminder of everything you need to know to successfully complete each workout. Use this as a checklist. If you're not sure about any point, go back and re-read the section of the book being referred to.

Have you planned in your diary what workout you will do and when?
Go back to the Introduction (page 16) for an 8-week sample diary. For ease you can simply copy this into your own diary.

Do you know what to do to warm up and cool down?
Go back and read "Dynamic Warm-up," page 30 and "Cool-down Stretches,"
page 108.

Are you clear about safety?
Go back and re-read "Safety and Technique considerations," pages 8–9.

Do you have all your equipment ready?
Go back and read "Clothing and Equipment," pages 12–13.

**Have you thought about which workouts can be used as substitutes if you
get bored or feel you need a new challenge?**
Go back and look at "How to Plan Your Workouts" in the Introduction,
pages 13–14.

Finally, and most important, do you know how to do each exercise?
Each workout will include 6 exercises plus a core strength exercise. All you
need to do is learn these 7 exercises thoroughly. Go back to the relevant
section for each exercise and slowly go through the motions of that exercise
paying particular attention to your technique and focus.

Core Workout–Beginners

This workout provides an important base to your program, providing you with a focused opportunity to develop your inner strength and flexibility.

Doing a dedicated core strength and length workout every week will improve your efficiency during your other workouts. It will focus on areas of the body that tend to get very tight or weak through general daily lifestyle habits. While this workout requires your fullest attention, you should find it a little easier to complete than other sessions. You can do your core strength and length workout on a rest day or do it on to the same day as another workout.

How to Get Going
- Follow each exercise as indicated in the relevant exercise section.
- Ensure you have all your equipment set up and ready to go.
- Take at least 5 minutes to warm up as indicated.
- Go through exercises 1–9 in succession, moving swiftly from one exercise to the next.
- Your intensity should be light to moderate—on a scale of 0–10 this is around 3–4. Go back and read the intensity guidelines to check that you are working at the correct level.
- Repeat the exercises a second time, always finishing on the calming stretches at the end.

To Warm Up: Go straight into your Dynamic Warm-up moves, repeating step one and spending at least 2 minutes on this before moving onto step 2.

The 20 Minute Workout: Each exercise will take you approximately 75 seconds to complete. This includes changeover time.

Exercise Order

1 The Secret Squeeze
2 The Dumb Waiter
3 Front Thigh And Hip Flexor Stretch
4 Wall Chest Stretch
5 On All Fours
6 Outer Chest Stretch
7 Foot Lifts
8 Deep Hip And Glute Stretch
9 Hamstring Stretch

Repeat 1–9

10 Back Rotation Stretch
11 Knee Hug

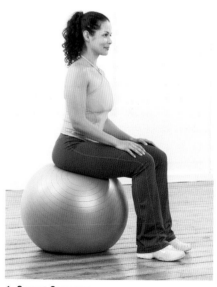

1 Secret Squeeze

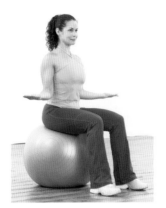
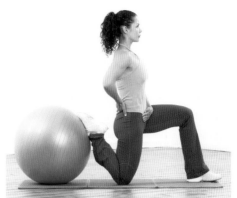

2 The Dumb Waiter

3 Front Thigh And Hip Flexor Stretch

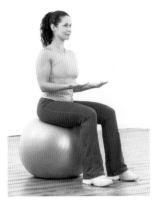
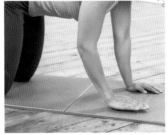
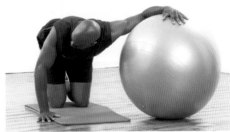

5 On All Fours

6 Outer Chest Stretch

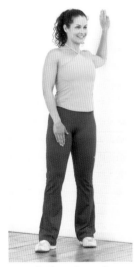
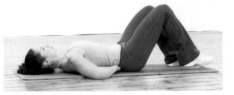
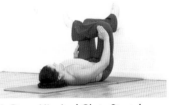

4 Wall Chest Stretch

7 Foot Lifts

8 Deep Hip And Glute Stretch

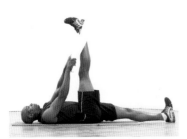
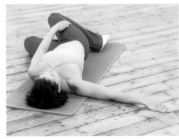
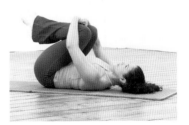

9 Hamstring Stretch

10 Back Rotation Stretch

11 Knee Hug

Core Workout–Advanced

To Warm Up: Go straight into your dynamic warm-up moves, repeating step one and spending at least 2 minutes on this before moving onto step 2.

The 20 Minute Workout: Each exercise will take you approximately 75 seconds to complete. This includes your changeover time.

Exercise Order

1 Posture Squat
2 Front Thigh And Hip Flexor Stretch
3 Outer Chest Stretch
4 Arrow Head
5 Press And Lift
6 Deep Chest Stretch
7 Knee Drops On The Step
8 Deep Hip And Glute Stretch
9 Hamstring Stretch

Repeat 1–9

10 Back Rotation Stretch
11 Knee Hug

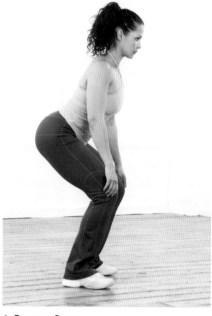

1 Posture Squat

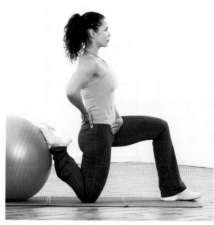

2 Front Thigh And Hip Flexor Stretch

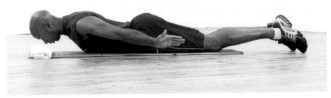

4 Arrow Head

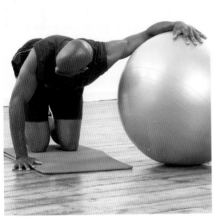

3 Outer Chest Stretch

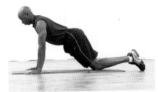

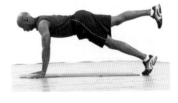

5 Press And Lift

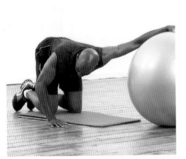

6 Deep Chest Stretch

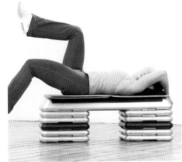

7 Knee Drops On The Step

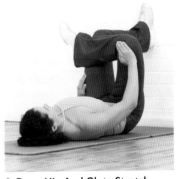

8 Deep Hip And Glute Stretch

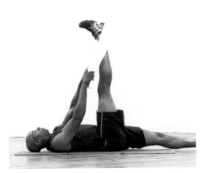

9 Hamstring Stretch

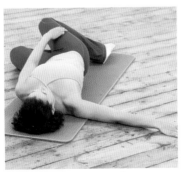

10 Back Rotation Stretch

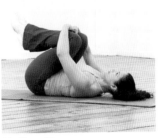

11 Knee Hug

129

Strength Circuit–Beginners

This workout is designed to increase your strength and lean muscle, boosting your metabolism and enabling you to burn extra fat, even when at rest.

The exercises have been designed to use your whole body rather than just one body part. This means you will use up more energy and burn more fat than in conventional strength training exercises.

How to Get Going:
- Follow each exercise as indicated in the exercise description section.
- Make sure you have all your equipment set up and ready to go.
- Take at least 5 minutes to warm up as indicated below
- Go through exercises 1–6 in succession, moving quickly from one exercise to the next.
- Your intensity should be moderate to moderately-hard. On a scale of 0–10 this is around 4–5. Go back and read your intensity guidelines to check that you are working at the correct level.
- Repeat the exercises a second time.
- Finish on a core exercise before moving on to your cool down stretches.

To Warm Up: Spend a minimum of 3 minutes on your first exercise, the Squat And Row, imitating the movement without using a band. Follow this with your Dynamic Warm-up moves.

The 20 Minute Workout: Each exercise will take you about 90 seconds to complete, including changeover time.

Exercise Order

1 Squat And Row
2 Forward Lunge
3 Seated Ball Press
4 Single Leg Glute Lift
5 Standing Tricep Extension
6 Towel Ab Curl

Repeat 1-6

Now Move On To Core Exercise: The Secret Squeeze.

To Cool Down: Finish with your cool-down stretches.

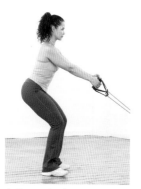
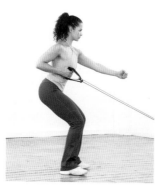
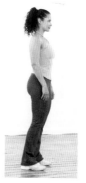
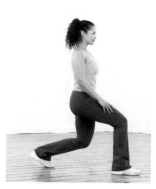

1 Squat And Row

2 Forward Lunge

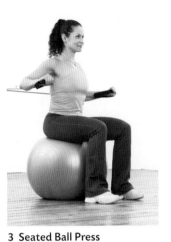

3 Seated Ball Press

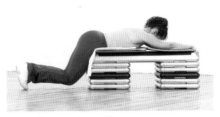

4 Single Leg Glute Lift

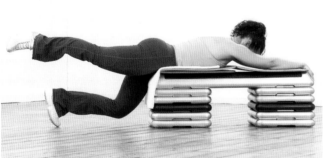

4 Single Leg Glute Lift

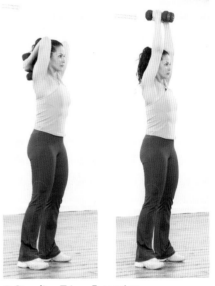

5 Standing Tricep Extension

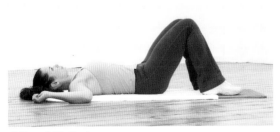

6 Towel Ab Curl

Strength Circuit–Advanced

To Warm-Up: Spend a minimum of three minutes on your first exercise, the Single Leg Squat and Row, imitating the movement without using a band. Follow this with your Dynamic Warm-up moves.

The 20 Minute Workout: Each exercise will take you approximately 90 seconds to complete. This includes your changeover time.

Exercise Order

1 Single Leg, Squat And Row
2 Jump Lunges
3 Lying Ball Press
4 Double Leg Glute Lift
5 Lying Ball Tricep Extension
6 Ab Curl On The Ball

Repeat 1–6

Now Move On To Core Exercise:
The Posture Squat.

To Cool Down: Finish with your cool-down stretches.

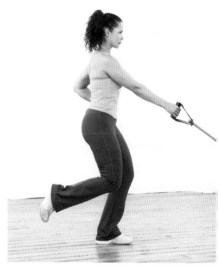

1 Single Leg, Squat And Row

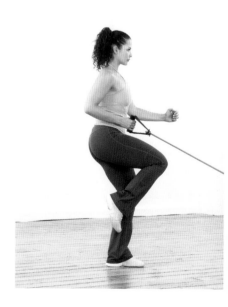

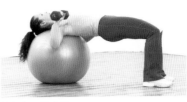

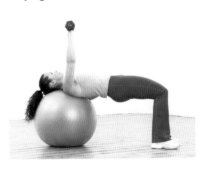

3 Lying Ball Press

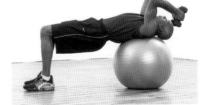

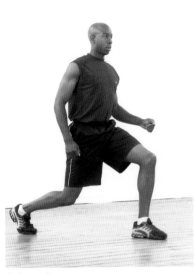
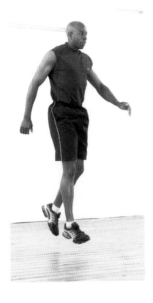

2 Jump Lunges

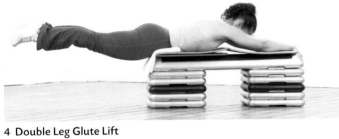

4 Double Leg Glute Lift

5 Lying Ball Tricep Extension

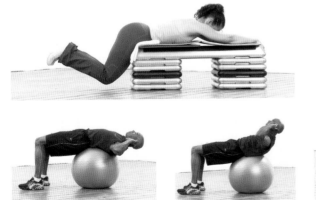
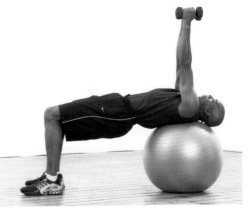

6 Ab Curl On The Ball

Cardio Circuit–Beginners

This exercise session is designed to work your heart and lungs, increasing your capacity to exercise for endurance.

Progressing this form of exercise to be able to work harder and for longer is key to improving your fat burning potential. You can also substitute these exercises for running or walking

How to Get Going
- Follow each exercise as indicated in the exercise description section.
- Make sure you have all your equipment set up and ready to go.
- Take at least 5 minutes to warm up as indicated below.
- Go through exercises 1–6 in succession, spending at least 3 minutes on each exercise.
- Check with your exercise descriptions to see if you need to change sides halfway through.
- Move quickly from one exercise to the next so that you spend no more than 20 minutes on this wotkout section.
- Your intensity should be moderate to hard. On a scale of 0–10 this is around 4–6. Go back and read your intensity guidelines to check that you are working at the correct level.
- Finish on a core exercise before moving on to your cool-down stretches.

To Warm-Up: Spend a minimum of 3 minutes on your first exercise, Step Ups, but on a lower step (6 inches). Follow this with your Dynamic Warm-up moves.

The 20 Minute Workout: Each exercise will take you approximately 3 mins to complete. This includes your changeover time.

Exercise Order

1 Step Ups
2 Rocking Horse
3 Front Kick
4 Knee Ups
5 Step In And Punch
6 Lunge Side And Back

Now Move On To Core Exercise: The Dumb Waiter.

To Cool Down: Finish with your cool-down stretches.

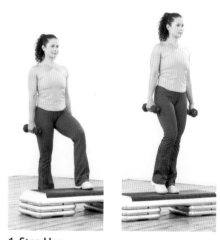

1 Step Ups

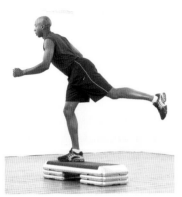

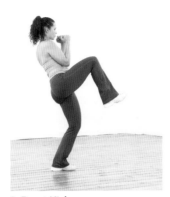

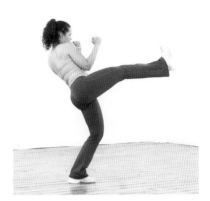

2 Rocking Horse

3 Front Kick

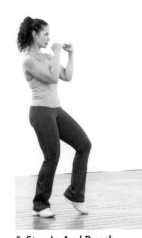

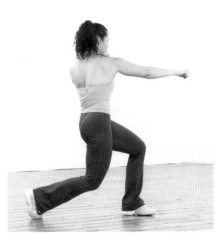

5 Step In And Punch

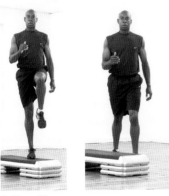

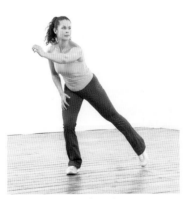

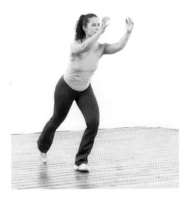

4 Knee Ups

6 Lunge Side And Back

Cardio Circuit–Advanced

To Warm Up: Spend a minimum of 3 minutes on your first exercise, Run Ups, but starting with step ups, moving onto slow run ups. Follow this with your Dynamic Warm-up moves.

The 20 Minute Workout: Each exercise will take you approximately 3 minutes and 30 seconds to complete. This includes your changeover time.

Exercise Order

1 Run Ups
2 Side Jump Lunges
3 Round House Kick
4 Knee Leap And lunge
5 Step In, Punch And Kick
6 Jump Up And Run Around

Now Move On To Core Exercise:
The Arrow Head.

To Cool Down: Finish with your cool-down stretches.

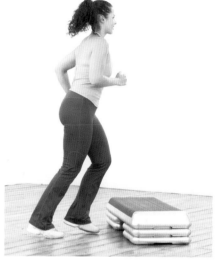

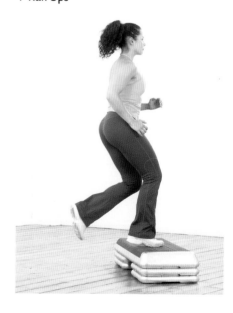

1 Run Ups

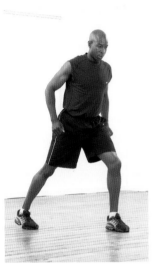
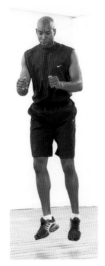

2 Side Jump Lunges

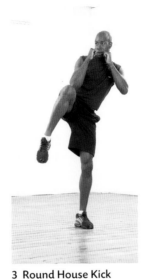
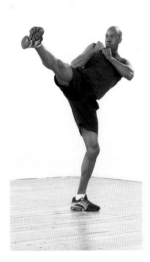

3 Round House Kick

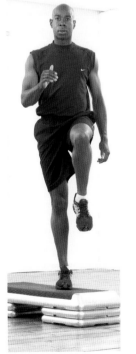
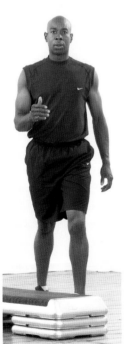

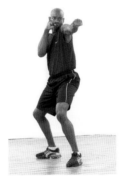
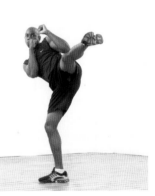

5 Step In, Punch And Kick

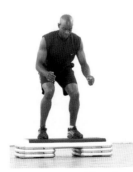
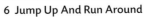

4 Knee Leap And lunge

6 Jump Up And Run Around

Step Circuit–Beginners

To strengthen your pelvic floor muscles, situated underneath your pelvis, supporting your lower torso and spine as well as helping to control your bladder and bowel.

Like the Cardio Circuit it will work your heart and lungs, increasing your capacity to exercise for endurance. Progressing to be able to work harder and for longer is key to improving your fat burning potential. You can also substitute these exercises with running or walking.

How to Get Going
- Follow each exercise as indicated in the exercise description section.
- Make sure that you have all your equipment set up and ready to go.
- Take at least 5 minutes to warm up as indicated.
- Go through exercises 1–6 in order spending at least 3 minutes on each exercise.
- Check with your exercise descriptions to see if you need to change sides halfway through.
- Move quickly from one exercise to the next so that you spend no more than 20 minutes on this section.
- Your intensity should be moderate to hard. On your scale of 0–10 this is around 4–6. Go back and read your intensity guidelines to check that you are working at the correct level.

To Warm Up: Spend a minimum of three minutes on your first exercise, Step Ups, but on a lower step (around 6 inches). Follow this by your Dynamic Warm-up moves.

The 20 Minute Workout: Each exercise will take you approximately 3 minutes to complete. This includes your changeover time.

Exercise Order

1 Step Ups
2 Rocking Horse
3 Knee Lifts On Step
4 Lunges Off The Back Of Step
5 Rocking Horse
6 Step Ups

Now Move On To Core Exercise: On All Fours.

To Cool Down: Finish with your cool-down stretches.

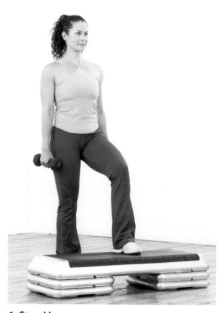

1 Step Ups

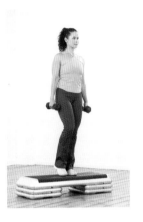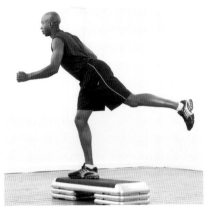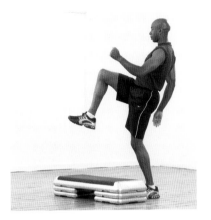

2 Rocking Horse

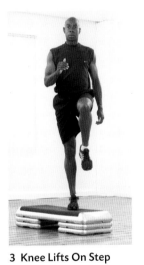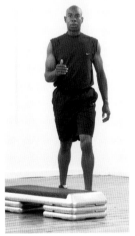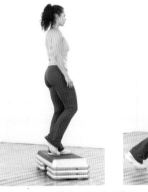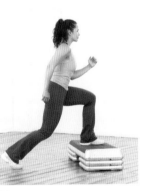

4 Lunges Off The Back Of Step

3 Knee Lifts On Step

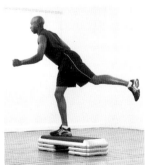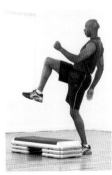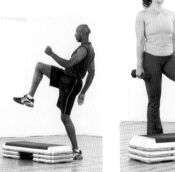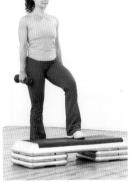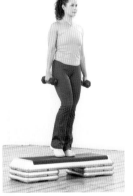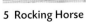

5 Rocking Horse

6 Step Ups

Step Circuit–Advanced

To Warm Up: Spend a minimum of 3 minutes on your first exercise, Run Ups, starting with step ups, moving onto slow run ups. Follow this by your Dynamic Warm-up moves.

The 20 Minute Workout: Each exercise will take you about 3 minutes and 30 seconds to complete, including changeover time.

Exercise Order

1 Run Ups
2 Lunges Off The Side Of Step
3 Jump Up And Run Around
4 Knee Leaps On The Step
5 Lunges Off The Side Of Step
6 Run Ups

Now Move On To Core Exercise: Press And Lift.

To Cool Down: Finish with your cool-down stretches.

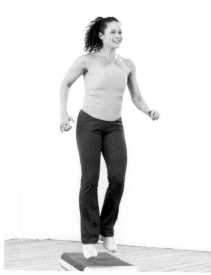

2 Lunges Off The Side Of Step

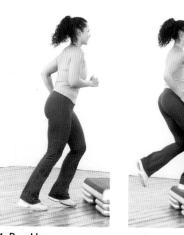

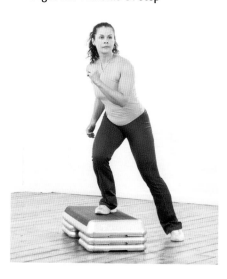

1 Run Ups

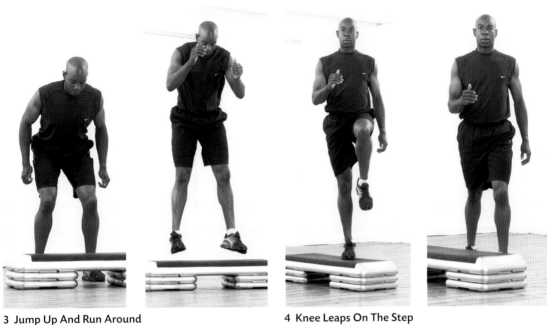

3 Jump Up And Run Around

4 Knee Leaps On The Step

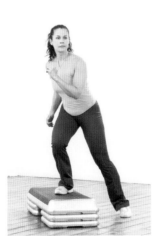

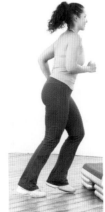

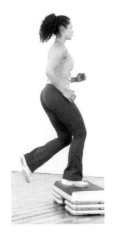

5 Lunges Off The Side Of Step

6 Run Ups

Mix It Session—Beginners

This exercise session is designed to work your heart and lungs while also providing strength benefits. Like the Cardio Circuit it is designed to keep your heart rate at a constant level.

This is done using strength exercises that are slightly harder to do in terms of intensity, enabling you to keep up a constant sweat and calorie burning effect.

How to Get Going
- Follow each exercise as indicated in the exercise description section.
- Make sure you have all your equipment set up and ready to go.
- Take at least 5 minutes to warm up as indicated below.
- Go through exercises 1–6 in succession, spending 2 minutes on each cardio exercise and 90 seconds on your on your strength exercises.
- Check with your exercise descriptions to see if you need to change sides halfway through. For this you will need to stop and change after either 1 minute or 40 seconds (see above).
- Your intensity should be moderate to hard. On your scale of 0–10 this is around 4–6. Go back and read your intensity guidelines to check that you are working at the correct level.

To Warm Up: Spend a minimum of 3 minutes on your first exercise, Step Ups, but on a lower step (6 inches). Follow this with your Dynamic Warm-up moves.

The 20 Minute Workout: Spend approximately 2 minutes on each cardio exercise and approx 90 seconds on each strength exercise. This includes your changeover time.

Exercise Order

1 Step Ups (cardio)
2 Squat And Row (strength)
3 Skip Jumps (cardio)
4 Wide Dumbbell Squat (strength)
5 Back Lunges Off The Step (cardio)
6 Seated Ball Press (strength)

Now Move on To Core Exercise: On All Fours.

To Cool Down: Finish with your cool-down stretches.

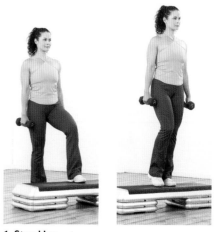

1 Step Ups

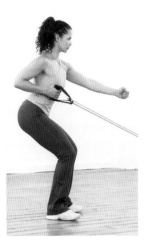

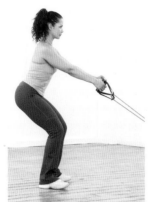

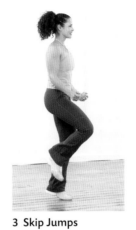

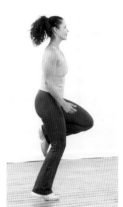

3 Skip Jumps

2 Squat And Row

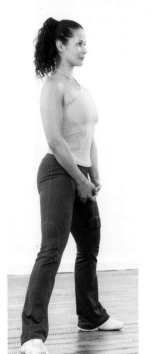

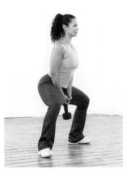

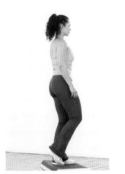

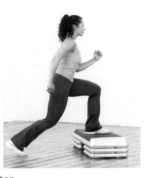

5 Back Lunges Off The Step

4 Wide Dumbbell Squat

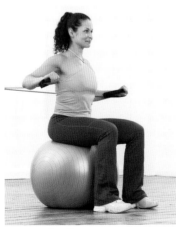

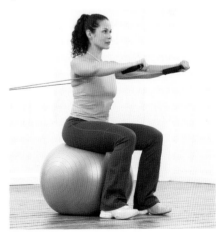

6 Seated Ball Press

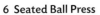

143

Mix It Session–Advanced

To Warm Up: Spend a minimum of 3 minutes on your first exercise, Run Ups, starting with step ups, moving onto slow run ups. Follow this with your Dynamic Warm-up moves.

The 20 Minute Workout: Spend approximately 2 minutes on each cardio exercise and approx 90 seconds each strength exercise. This includes your changeover time.

Exercise Order

1 Run Ups (cardio)
2 Single Leg Squat and Row (strength)
3 Lunges Off The Side Of Step (cardio)
4 Lying Ball Press (strength)
5 High Step Ups (cardio)
6 Lunge Back And Lift (strength)

Now Move on To Core Exercise: Posture Squat.

To Cool Down: Finish with your cool-down stretches.

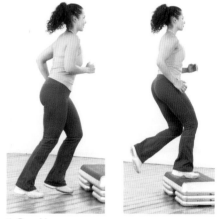

1 Run Ups

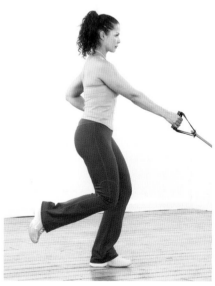

2 Single Leg Squat and Row

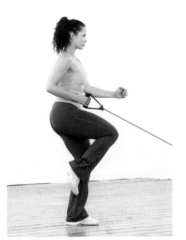
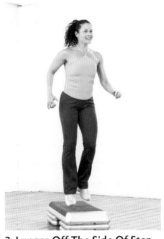
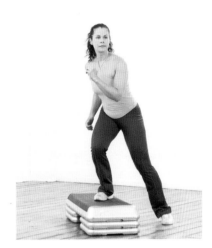

3 Lunges Off The Side Of Step

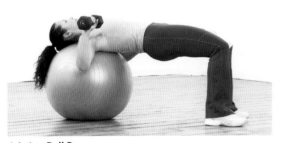
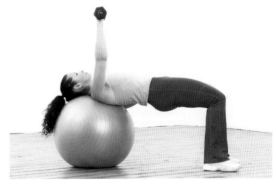

4 Lying Ball Press

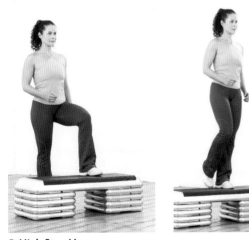
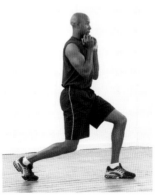
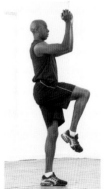

5 High Step Ups

6 Lunge Back And Lift

Outdoor Cross Trainer– Beginners

Like the Fat Burner Mix It session, your Outdoor Cross Trainer session is designed to work the heart and lungs, while providing strength benefits.

Instead of working inside, you are going to use the outdoors to replicate your strength and cardio moves.

How to Get Going
- Follow each exercise as indicated in the exercise description section while taking note of the points below for adapting your moves for outside.
- For equipment you will need your exercise band. Attach your band to tree branches for high positions, bench legs for low positions, and fences or bench seats for mid positions.
- Instead of using a ball you can sit or kneel against a park bench and attach your band around the back of the bench or to a bench leg.
- You will also need to look for a bench or series of steps that you can step up and down on (either go to your local park or set up your steps).
- You will also need a circuit or route to run or walk around. This needs to take you approximately 3 minutes. Try using a section of a park, for example, around a lake or the perimeter of a field.
- Take at least 5 minutes to warm up as indicated below.
- Go through exercises 1–6 spending 2 minutes on each cardio exercise and 90 seconds on the strength exercises.
- Check with your exercise descriptions if you need to change sides halfway through. For this you will need to stop and change after 1 minute or 40 seconds (see above).

- Your intensity should be moderate to hard. On your scale of 0–10 this is around 4–6. Go back and read your intensity guidelines to check that you are working at the correct level.
- You will find it easier to follow your Short Stretch routine if finishing your workout outside.

To Warm Up: Spend a minimum of 3 minutes on your first exercise, Power Walk, but at a lower intensity. Begin by gently walking and gradually build up. Follow this by your Dynamic Warm-up moves.

The 20 Minute Workout: Spend approximately 2 minutes on each cardio exercise and approximately 90 seconds on each strength exercise. This includes your changeover time.

Exercise Order

1 Power Walk or Run and Walk
2 Squat And Row
3 Skip Jumps
4 Forward Lunge
5 Step Ups
6 Seated Rotation And Lift

Now Move on To Core Exercise: On All Fours.

To Cool Down: Finish with your cool-down stretches.

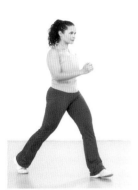
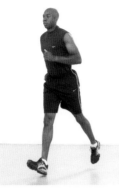

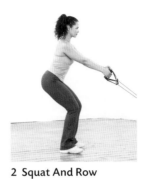
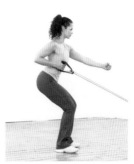

2 Squat And Row

1 Power Walk or Run and Walk

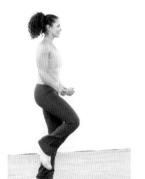
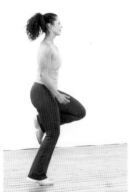

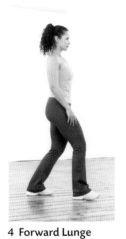
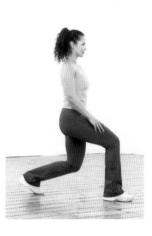

3 Skip Jumps

4 Forward Lunge

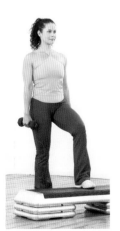
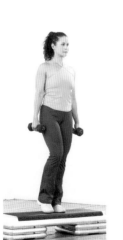

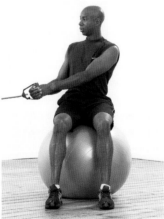
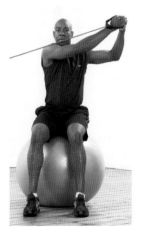

5 Step Ups

6 Seated Rotation And Lift

Outdoor Cross Trainer– Advanced

To Warm Up: Spend a minimum of 3 minutes on your first exercise, Power Walk or Run, but at a lower intensity. Begin by gently walking and gradually build up. Follow this with your Dynamic Warm-up moves.

The 20 Minute Workout: Spend approximately 2 minutes on each cardio exercise and approx 90 seconds on each strength exercise. This includes your changeover time.

Exercise Order

1 Power Walk or Run (cardio)
2 Single Leg Squat and Row (strength)
3 Run Ups (cardio)
4 Lunge Jumps (strength)
5 High Step Ups (cardio)
6 Squat, Rotate And Lift (strength)

Now Move on To Core Exercise: Press and Lift.

To Cool Down: Finish with your cool-down stretches.

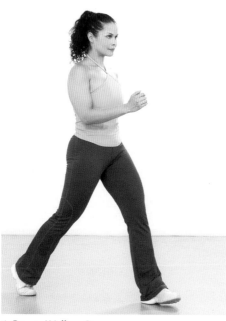
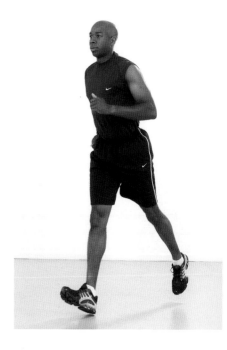

1 Power Walk or Run

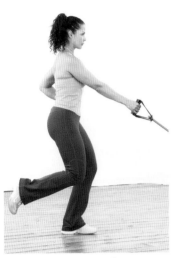

2 Single Leg Squat and Row

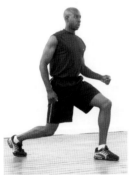

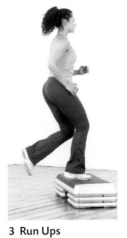

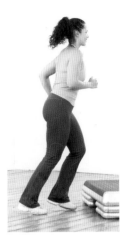

3 Run Ups

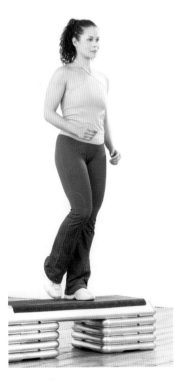

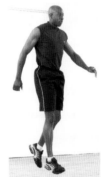

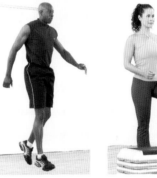

4 Lunge Jumps

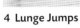

5 High Step Ups

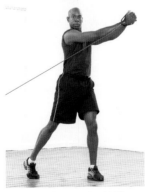

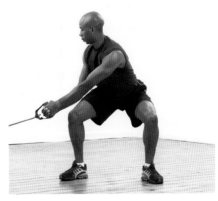

6 Squat, Rotate And Lift

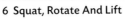

149

Interval Session—Beginners

This session differs to the others in that, rather than working up toward a sustainable intensity, your aim is to do short cardiovascular bursts of high intensity exercise, followed by recovery periods of equal length.

By doing this workout you will greatly improve your fitness levels which, in the long run, will help to boost your metabolism and increase your ability to burn fat.

How to Get Going
- Follow each exercise as indicated in the exercise description section.
- Make sure you have all your equipment set up and ready to go.
- Take at least 5 minutes to warm up as indicated below.
- Go through exercises 1–6 in succession, spending 2 minutes on each exercise, then repeat the exercises a second time, spending 1 minute on each.
- Check with your exercise descriptions if you need to change sides halfway through.
- You may find in your strength exercises that, to keep to the time restraints, you need to alter the speed or decrease the number of repetitions. This is fine. Remember that strength exercises are a recovery phase, doing enough to keep you in the lower regions of your fat burning zone but not so much that you can't recover.
- With your cardio bursts, aim to work a little harder than in your Cardio Circuit or Mix it sessions. Do this by increasing your pace or using the exercise progressions while still using good technique.
- For your cardio bursts you should be working hard, at around 6–7 on your intensity scale of 0–10. Go back and read intensity guidelines to check you

are working at the correct level.
- If you find that you are not recovering sufficiently before moving onto your next high intensity burst, you are working too hard and need to ease off the pace.

To Warm Up: Spend a minimum of 3 minutes on your first exercise, Skip Jumps, working very slowly and with small skipping moves. Follow this with your Dynamic Warm-up moves.

The 20 Minute Workout: For your first round spend 2 minutes on each cardio exercise and 2 minutes on each strength exercise. Shorten this to 1 minute on each for your second round. This includes your changeover time.

Exercise Order

1 Skip Jumps (cardio burst)
2 Seated Rotate And Lift (strength recovery)
3 Squat And Jump (cardio burst)
4 Single Lat Pull Down (strength recovery)
5 Side To Side Leaps (cardio burst)
6 Foot Lifts (strength recovery)

Repeat 1–6 spending 1 minute on each

Now Move on To Core Exercise: Dumb Waiter.

To Cool Down: Finish with your cool-down stretches.

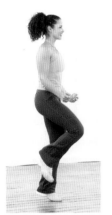
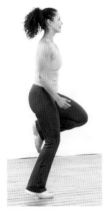
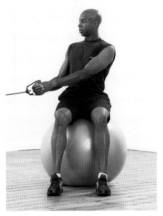
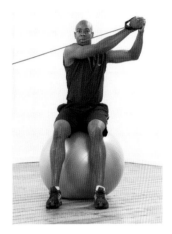

1 Skip Jumps

2 Seated Rotate And Lift

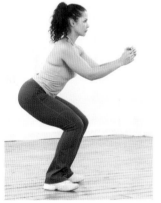
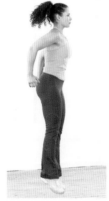
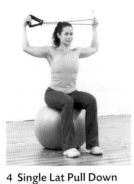
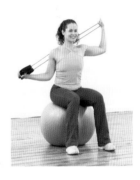

4 Single Lat Pull Down

3 Squat And Jump

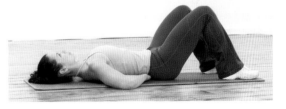

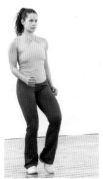
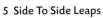
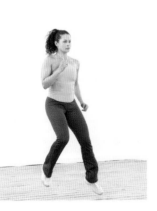
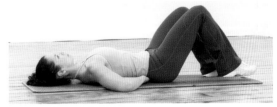

5 Side To Side Leaps

6 Foot Lifts

Interval Session–Advanced

To Warm Up: Spend a minimum of 3 minutes on your first exercise, Run Ups, but start with step ups, moving onto slow run ups. Follow this with your Dynamic Warm-up moves.

The 20 Minute Workout: For your first round spend 2 minutes on each cardio exercise and 2 minutes on each strength exercise. Shorten this to 1 minute on each for your second round. This includes your changeover time.

Exercise Order

1 Run Ups (cardio burst)
2 Squat, Rotate, And Lift (strength recovery)
3 Ski Jumps (cardio burst)
4 Straight Arm Pull Down (strength recovery)
5 Leap Over The Step (cardio burst)
6 Knee Drops On The Step (strength recovery)

Repeat 1–6 spending 1 minute on each

Now Move on To Core Exercise: The Arrow head.

To Cool Down: Finish with your cool-down stretches.

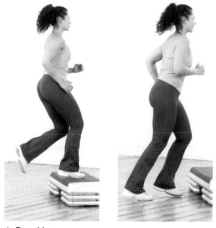

1 Run Ups

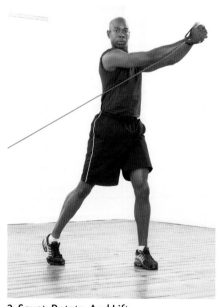

2 Squat, Rotate, And Lift

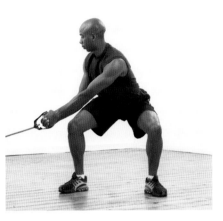
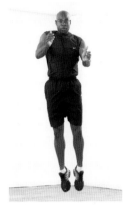
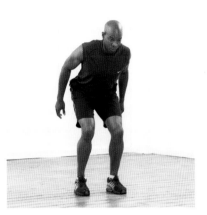

3 Ski Jumps

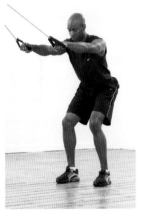
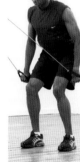
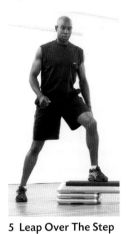
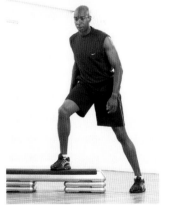

4 Straight Arm Pull Down

5 Leap Over The Step

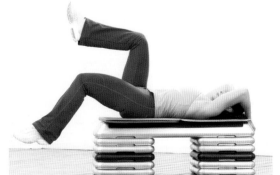

6 Knee Drops On The Step

Outdoor Interval—Beginners

Like your indoor interval session, your aim is to do short cardiovascular bursts of high intensity exercise, followed by recovery periods of equal length.

By doing this workout you will greatly improve your fitness levels which, in the long run, will help to boost your metabolism and increase your ability to burn fat.

How to Get Going

- Follow each exercise as indicated in the exercise description section while taking note of the points below for adapting your moves outside.
- You will need to take your exercise band. Attach your band to tree branches for high positions, bench legs for low positions, and fences or bench seats for mid positions.
- You will need to look for a park bench or a series of steps that you can step up and down on. You find them in your local park or set up your step.
- You will need a circuit or route. This needs to take you about 3 minutes.
- Go through exercises 1–6 in succession, spending 2 minutes on each exercise, then repeat the exercises a second time, 1 minute on each.
- You may find in the strength exercises that to keep to the time restraints, you need to alter the speed or decrease number of repetitions. This is fine. Remember that strength exercises are a recovery phase, doing enough to keep you in the lower regions of your fat burning zone but allowing you to recover.
- With your cardio bursts, aim to work a little harder than in your Cardio Circuit or Mix It sessions: around 6–7 on your intensity scale of 0–10.
- If you find that you are not recovering well before moving onto

your next high intensity burst you are working too hard and need to ease off the pace.
- If finishing outside, it may be easier to do a short stretch routine.

To Warm Up: Spend a minimum of 3 minutes on your first exercise Power Walk or Run, but at a lower intensity. Begin by gently walking and gradually build up. Follow this by your Dynamic Warm-up moves.

The 20 Minute Workout: For your first round spend 2 minutes on each cardio exercise and 2 minutes on each strength exercise. Shorten this to 1 minute on each for your second round. This includes your changeover time.

Exercise Order

1 Run or Run and Walk (cardio burst)
2 Seated Ball Press: try using a bench (strength recovery)
3 Squat And Jump (cardio burst)
4 Single Lat Pull Down (strength recovery)
5 Side To Side Leaps (cardio burst)
6 Foot Lifts (strength recovery)

Repeat 1–6 spending 1 minute on each

Now Move on To Core Exercise: Dumb Waiter.

To Cool Down: Finish with your cool-down stretches.

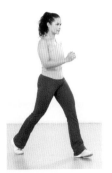
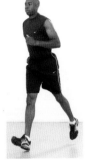

1 Run or Run and Walk

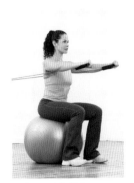

2 Seated Ball Press

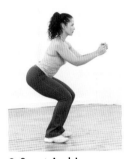
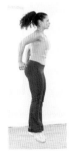
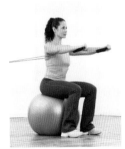

3 Squat And Jump

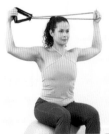
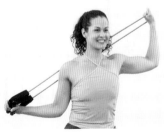

4 Single Lat Pull Down

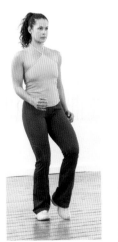

5 Side To Side Leaps

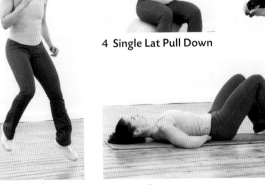
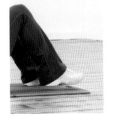

6 Foot Lifts

Outdoor Interval–Advanced

To Warm Up: Spend a minimum of 3 minutes on your first exercise Power Walk or Run, but at a lower intensity. Begin by walking and gradually build up. Follow this by your Dynamic Warm-up moves.

The 20 Minute Workout: For your first round spend 2 minutes on each cardio exercise and 2 minutes on each strength exercise. Shorten this to 1 minute on each for your second round. This includes your changeover time.

Exercise Order

1 Run or Power Walk (cardio burst)
2 Squat, Rotate, And Lift (strength recovery)
3 Ski Jumps (cardio burst)
4 Straight Arm Pull Down (strength recovery)
5 High Steps Ups (cardio burst)
6 Knee Drops On The Step.(You can use a bench) (strength recovery)

Repeat 1–6 spending 1 minute on each

Now Move on To Core Exercise: The Press and Lift.

To Cool Down: Finish with your cool-down stretches.

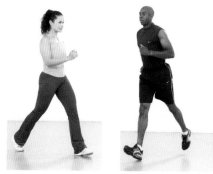

1 Run or Power Walk

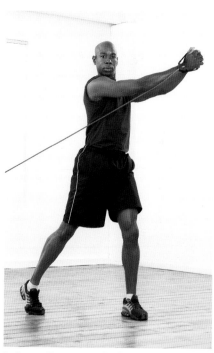

2 Squat, Rotate, And Lift

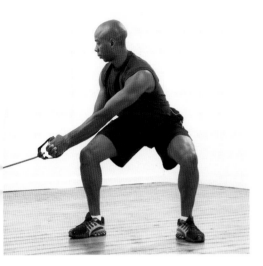
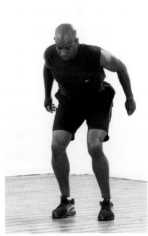
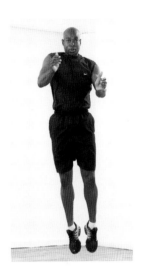

3 Ski Jumps

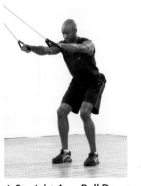
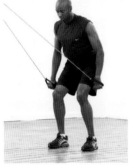
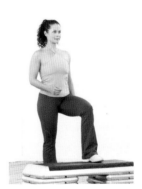
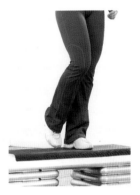

4 Straight Arm Pull Down

5 High Steps Ups

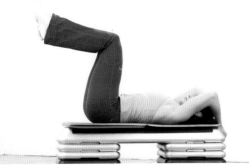
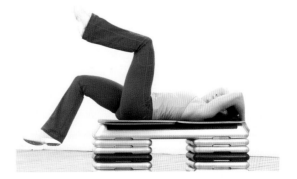

6 Knee Drops On The Step

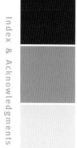

Index

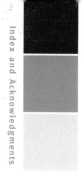

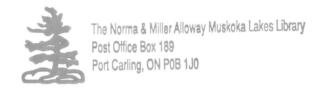
Acknowledgments

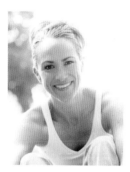

I would like to thank members of my personal training team, Stan and Kim for being such great models for the book, and Michelle who modeled for the front cover. I would also like to thank my husband who tirelessly put up with my early morning tappings at the computer and my little baby who, yet to be born, had to put up with his mother's long working hours at 8 months pregnant!

Jane Wake

Models: Kim James and Stan Blair
Photographer: Eddie Macdonald

All images © Chrysalis Image Library/Eddie Macdonald apart from the following:

© Digital Stock 6 (center)
© Stockbyte 6 (left), 6 (right), 7
© Chrysalis Image Library 8

Chrysalis Books Group Plc is committed to respecting the intellectual property rights of others. We have therefore taken all reasonable efforts to ensure that the reproduction of all content on these pages is done with the full consent of copyright owners. If you are aware of any unintentional omissions please contact the company directly so that any necessary corrections may be made for future editions.